The Creative Side of Experimentation

Personal Perspectives From Leading Researchers in Motor Control, Motor Development, and Sport Psychology

Conrad Wesley Snyder, Jr., PhD
Ohio University

Bruce Abernethy, PhD
University of Queensland

Editors

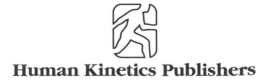

Human Kinetics Publishers

This book is offered as a memorial to Dr. Warren D. Walsh, University of Queensland, who typified the creative and curious scientist that we hope this book may aid in developing.

Library of Congress Cataloging-in-Publication Data

The Creative side of experimentation : personal perspectives from
  leading researchers in motor control, motor development, and sport
  psychology / Conrad Wesley Snyder, editor, Bruce Abernethy, editor.
    p.   cm.
  Includes bibliographical references and index.
  ISBN 0-87322-376-4
  1. Motor ability--Research--Methodology.   2. Motor learning-
  -Research--Methodology.   3. Sports--Psychological aspects--Research-
  -Methodology.   4. Psychological research personnel--Biography.
  I. Snyder, Conrad Wesley, 1943-   . II. Abernethy, Bruce, 1958-   .
  QP301.C66   1992
  612.7'6'072--dc20   92-6234
                                                                           CIP

ISBN: 0-87322-376-4

Acquisitions Editor: Rick Frey, PhD   Indexer: Barbara Cohen
Developmental Editor: Holly Gilly   Production Director: Ernie Noa
Managing Editor: Moyra Knight   Typesetting and Page Layout: Sandra Meier
Assistant Editor: Laura Bofinger   Text Design: Keith Blomberg
Copyeditor: Julie Anderson   Cover Design: Linda Brown
Proofreader: Julia Anderson   Printer: Braun-Brumfield

Printed in the United States of America

10 9 8 7 6 5 4 3 2 1

Human Kinetics Publishers   *Europe Office:*
Box 5076, Champaign, IL 61825-5076   Human Kinetics Publishers (Europe) Ltd.
1-800-747-4457   P.O. Box IW14
                                         Leeds LS16 6TR
Canada Office: England
Human Kinetics Publishers, Inc.   0532-781708
P.O. Box 2503
Windsor, ON N8Y 4S2   *Australia Office:*
1-800-465-7301 (in Canada only)   Human Kinetics Publishers
                                         P.O. Box 80
                                         Kingswood 5062
                                         South Australia
                                         374-0433

Contents

About the Editors

Drs. Wes Snyder, Jr. and Bruce Abernethy have more than 30 years' combined experience in human movement research and instruction. Their extensive backgrounds make them uniquely qualified to edit *The Creative Side of Experimentation*.

Wes Snyder is the director of the Center for Higher Education and International Programs at Ohio University, where he is also a professor of applied behavioral science and educational leadership. Specializing in research design, he has taught in Australia and Africa as well as the United States. He has done extensive research in human movement, psychology of affect, international development and program evaluation, and sociology of organizations.

Dr. Snyder earned his PhD from the University of Pennsylvania with a dissertation on measurement, evaluation, and techniques of experimental research. He is a member of the American Psychological Association, the American Sociological Association, and the Psychometric Society.

Bruce Abernethy is professor and head of the Department of Human Movement Studies at the University of Queensland in Australia and an active researcher and teacher in motor learning and control. Currently the editor-in-chief of the *Australian Journal of Science and Medicine in Sport*, he is also an editorial board member of the *International Journal of Sport Psychology* and an occasional reviewer for such journals as *Human Movement Science* and the *Research Quarterly for Exercise and Sport*.

Dr. Abernethy earned his PhD from the University of Otago in New Zealand with a dissertation on expertise in perception and action. He is a member of the North American Society for the Psychology of Sport and Physical Activity and the International Society of Sport Psychology.

Preface

Questions regarding how motor skills are acquired and controlled, how they are influenced by maturational change, and how they are modified by personal or situational variables are the focal interest of theoreticians and practitioners in the movement sciences. Knowledge related to these questions has been acquired by researchers applying the methodological procedures and practices of a myriad of established scientific disciplines, including physiology, physics, mathematics, computer science, and psychology. Contemporary theoretical notions of human motor control, for example, have their roots in the engineering sciences, with the control systems analogies; in mathematics and computer sciences, with information-processing concepts; in physics, with dynamical systems models; in the neurosciences, in terms of neural circuitry hypotheses; and in the applied databases of many other fields, such as ergonomics, robotics, linguistics, and rehabilitative medicine. Although researchers who study the problems posed by human action have varied backgrounds, the dominant parentage has nevertheless been experimental psychology. The ancestral links with experimental psychology remain intact in the areas of study today delineated as motor learning and control, motor development, and sport and exercise psychology.

What This Book Is All About

In this book we examine how experimentation aids in our understanding of motor learning and control, motor development, and sport and exercise psychology. In Part I, we discuss experimentation in general terms, highlighting what uniquely characterizes an experiment and sets it aside from other human experiences and observations. We discuss different types of experimentation and the steps that are typically involved in the experimentation process, noting that experimentation is a much more creative and less rule-bound activity than is typically acknowledged. We emphasize, in particular, the need to understand the personal characteristics, beliefs, and cognitions of experimenters themselves in order to fully understand how experimentation proceeds in practice; we draw attention to how much of this essential insight into experimentation is lost in the formal reports of published research and is left unacknowledged in traditional texts on experimentation.

Parts II, III, and IV provide first-person insights into the experimentation process through autobiographical accounts of experimentation by noted researchers in the motor learning and control, motor development, and sport and exercise psychology fields. In chapters 2 through 13 these noted researchers, chosen because of their contributions to the development of knowledge in each of these fields, openly discuss their career developments and their pivotal experimental works, providing unique insights into their motives, hunches, biases, and cognitions as they use the experiment as a means of better understanding the nature of human action. For each field of human action research, we provide brief overviews of the central historical developments and contemporary issues and trends in the field. A short descriptive portrait of each researcher is included to place the researcher's contributions in an appropriate historical context. In keeping with the themes developed in Part I, these autobiographies show experimentation as a dynamic, interactive, and creative human endeavor through which carefully planned and controlled observations can give rise to deeper understanding of complex phenomena. Our rationale for including personalized accounts of the experimentation experiences of eminent human action researchers is both to convey the spirit of each experimenter's enthusiasm and accomplishments and to provide the reader with insight into the means by which critical decisions in the experimentation process are made. We believe that this information—which is lost in standard scientific reports of experimentation, but which is clearly an integral part of the experimentation process—is invaluable for better understanding how current methodological approaches and design prescriptions to the study of human action have emerged.

The authors of the autobiographical chapters are well-known researchers who have contributed significantly to understanding in their fields. Other researchers (including women, we hasten to add) were invited and could not participate. There are many other researchers of eminence that could have been included, but we didn't have room to include them all. The authors included in this book represent both the "hard" and "soft" experimental preferences in approach. They reflect varied backgrounds and influences on their careers, and they illustrate past and present research styles in the movement sciences. They are exemplars of the "family of experimentalists" in the movement sciences and are useful case studies for researchers just beginning their careers in experimentation in the human action fields. The achievements of the noted experimentalists result from (of course) their talents and sensitivities but also from their interest in learning, their preparation in and understanding of their areas of interest, their perseverance in the pursuit of knowledge, some serendipity (being in the right place at the right time and perhaps trying the right things), and their facility with experimentation. There is much, we believe, to be learned from their personal reflections on experimentation.

Part V attempts to synthesize the autobiographical accounts of experimentation provided in chapters 2 through 13 into a description of the skills and approaches that typify expert experimentation. Although there are few hard-and-fast rules to success in experimentation, and the diversity within the backgrounds, methods, and styles of successful experimenters is overwhelming, some commonalities nevertheless emerge that have important implications for the would-be experimentalist. Expert experimenters share many attributes in common with experts from other cognitive tasks, especially with respect to their abilities to structure the knowledge within their fields and to see links and relationships that are not evident to the lesser skilled. In particular, expert experimenters appear to make their greatest impact upon their fields by introducing new ways of looking at old problems, frequently by importing to their fields concepts and methods developed and utilized in other seemingly unrelated fields. We discuss in Part V not only the characteristics of expert experimenters but also the implications of these characteristics for the preparation of a new generation of experimenters who are capable of extending the bounds of knowledge about human action beyond its current limits. We also reiterate in Part V the view of experimentation as a dynamic human endeavor influenced by individual differences in creativity, insight, and modes of thinking, rather than a constrained, mechanistic pursuit (as "cookbook" recitations of the scientific method would have us believe).

How to Use This Book

There are at least three ways to use this book—as an introduction to the experimentation process, as an insight into expertise in experimentation, or as an adjunct to graduate coursework in motor learning and control, motor development, or sport and exercise psychology. If you are using the book primarily to learn about how the experimentation process works in practice, carefully read chapter 1 to gain an understanding of the traditional view of experimentation and the extent of subjective influences at all stages of the experimentation process. Then carefully peruse the autobiographical accounts, noting the steps the experimenters took and the kinds of decisions they made in performing pivotal research. Use the autobiographical accounts to share in the experimenters' senses of achievement but also to share the frustrations and concerns that researchers must continually overcome in order to establish successful, progressive lines of research. Note how each experimenter's personal insights and cognitions play an important role throughout the experimentation process and how these subjective aspects of the experimentation process infrequently appear in formal reports of experiments. Compare one or more of the autobiographical reports with the original published reports of the same experiments to see how the published reports bear only limited resemblance to the actual genesis and development of the original research idea.

If you are using the book to gain insight into what it takes to be an expert experimenter, then in reading Parts II through IV look for commonalities in background education and experience, in approaches to solving problems, in strategies for experimental design, and in personal traits and attributes. In perusing the brief sections on the history of and trends and issues in the human action fields, note how many different theoretical views are possible and how each is, in a sense, a prisoner of its own particular era; yet note how from time to time, ideas and methods are introduced by researchers that allow the field to progress beyond its current confines into a new era of understanding. Try, in reading the autobiographies of successful researchers, to tease out what you perceive to be the important characteristics of those experimenters who generated new insights where previously only confusion existed (i.e., who generated order out of chaos), and compare your observations with our synthesis on expertise in experimentation presented in chapter 14.

If you are using the book to complement formal coursework in any of the human action fields, read first the sectional summaries on the history of and trends and current issues in your field of interest; then read the brief introductions to each of the contributing authors. These introductions cite the contributions and theoretical positions of the individual experimenters within the broader context of the historical and contemporary development of the field. These sections alone may provide a valuable organizational framework upon which to assemble and evaluate new knowledge and upon which to design your own experiments. Follow this by reading the autobiographies of each of the four noted researchers within your field of interest. Compare these autobiographical accounts of their research with their formal published work and observe both the degree of creativity and the unique situational constraints that fashioned each experimenter's work. Learn from the attributes and strategies of successful experimenters in your field (chapter 14 may help in this regard) so that you gain a better feel for both the personal history of your field and the kind of experiments and experimenters needed to continue to advance the field.

Acknowledgments

An individual's ideas are in some ways unique, but, fortunately for us, in most ways they are more common or at least can be usefully constructed to be so. In this book, the various authors have invoked the ideas and comments of many philosophers and researchers, and we acknowledge the debt to those who laid the scientific foundation for understanding human action. Glimpses of precedent thought were provided to create a sense of history and to hopefully encourage the search for primary sources. We trust our constructions of the world of experimentation and the larger world of science do these earlier ideas justice.

We also owe a debt of gratitude to our loved ones (Debbie, Heather, Joclynn, Kirsten, and our parents and friends) and to the colleagues whose work we particularly respect (the contributors to this book). Kathy Blaine, Shirley Greer, and Judy Land helped significantly in entering the chapter text, and figures were produced using Innovative Data Design's MacDraft and Aldus's PageMaker. We appreciate Rainer Martens's patience, as we illustrated once again that "things take more time than they do." Richard Frey, our acquisitions editor, steered us through many modifications in size and scope for the book (in fact, we have another book left over!). Holly Gilly, our developmental editor, gave us a target and helped us aim our efforts; her assistance was invaluable. (She even managed to have a baby during our collaboration—we often joked that young Benjamin would probably be reading the proofs if we didn't soon get it right.) Moyra Knight, our managing editor, kept track of the details and made sure the pieces came together. Debbie and Bruce also had a new baby, Mitchell, just as we finished. So we are pleased to have completed this book for our expanding audience.

Part I

Experimentation:
An Introduction

Observation is more than noting what meets the eye and experimentation is more than an interesting exploration through personal experiences, although a sharp eye and an inquisitive nature are nevertheless important in experimentation. Chapter 1 examines the formalities of experimentation, emphasizing that the process of experimentation is much richer and more dynamic than we typically recognize and acknowledge. The chapter first examines the essential elements that constitute an experiment, highlighting directed observation and notions of control as necessary conditions. Next, the chapter presents contrasting views on how the experiment contributes, or should contribute, to scientific knowledge. The traditional top-down or theory-driven approach to experimentation is presented and then contrasted with alternative types of experimentation in which the knowledge-generation cycle is initiated not by a refined theory but rather by either new data (bottom-up experimentation) or new technology (method-driven experimentation). Next, the chapter briefly considers the dynamics of arbitrarily defined stages in the experimentation process and introduces key notions pertaining to cycles of normal and revolutionary science in the advancement of knowledge and pertaining to the extent of decision making facing the experimenter throughout each stage of the experimentation process. Finally, the chapter highlights the impacts of the personal characteristics, beliefs, biases, and cognitions of the experimenter upon the experimentation process; a rationale is established for the importance of inspecting, autobiographically, the important cognitions of eminent experimenters in the human action field. Throughout this chapter, and indeed throughout the book, experimentation is portrayed as an exciting, dynamic process rather than a passive, mechanistic one. The experimenter's imagination and innovation are presented as major contributors to the generation of knowledge through science.

Chapter 1

Fundamentals of Experimentation

Bruce Abernethy
Conrad W. Snyder, Jr.

In order to discuss experimentation we first define it by identifying those characteristics that set it apart from other human activities.

What Is an Experiment?

Experimentation is a planned set of observations by which we explore (conceptually) discrete components of our experiences. We can look at human activities and explore the complexities of humanity without experimenting, and we can experience the continuous flow of life whether or not our personal constructs are given the precise boundaries of formal variables. But experiments enhance our fleeting and singular understandings. They provide a chance for us to try out and reflect upon our theoretical speculations within the context of "controlled" human experience. Experiments are one way in which we can analyze our world of experience so that we can share our conceptual understandings with others through empirical tests of initial or refined speculations. Experimentation in motor learning and control, motor development, and sport and exercise psychology provides a way for us to understand more about the processes and events that underlie our personal experiences of actions routinely performed and observed in the home, in the work place, and in the settings of competitive sport and recreational activities.

The Importance of Directed Observation

Experiments differ from normal experience in a number of fundamental ways. First, an experiment constitutes a special experience because of its

3

reliance on *directed observation*. In everyday experience we see much of what goes on around us, but we do not apply our complete intelligence to deal with it, we do not ponder its minutiae, and we do not conscientiously examine its relationships. In experimentation, we carefully and thoroughly scrutinize the observed event and apply our observational and intellectual skills to the fullest in an attempt to understand the studied phenomenon.

To What Extent Is Observer Objectivity Possible?

A second requirement of experimentation, which is frequently listed in traditional introductory texts on the scientific method, is that not only should the experimenter's observation of the event be extremely careful and precise, but also pristine and unsullied, uninfluenced by the experimenter's personal bias or subjectivity. For these criteria to be met, two experimenters carefully observing the same event need to report the same perceptual experience of the event. This would give rise to intersubjective agreement, a notion carried over into the philosophy of science from the reign of logical positivism. Such a requirement upon an experiment is, however, not only unrealistic and perhaps impossible but also unnecessarily constraining on the creative and interpretative skills of the individual experimenter and in turn upon the development of knowledge.

Even if we agree with another independent observer about what we see, we can still be wrong, as in the case of an illusion created masterfully and intentionally by a magician. In an experimental program, verification will eventually be open to replicated experiences and public verdicts. However, in a particular experiment, all we can ask is that the experimenter try to be neutral, unbiased from personal hopes and overzealous expectations. Scriven (1972) calls this *qualitative objectivity*. Qualitative objectivity is concerned with the quality of the observation in an experiment, not the number of observers or their agreement. Such a notion is necessary in a given experiment, because one person with singularly astute observational skills can observe what others may miss! Just as one careful observer may uncover how a magician produces a given illusion while hundreds of other observers report common but incorrect perceptions of the same event, careful and creative experimenters may find better ways of explaining given experimental observations than do the majority of experimenters. We will see later in this chapter how new ways of looking at research problems that are in conflict with the favored view of the time are indeed essential for the advancement of understanding in any given field of science.

In directed observation during experimentation, as in all aspects of day-to-day perception, what is seen varies substantially from one observer to the next. In standard laboratory studies of perception, the perceptual experiences reported by observers vary according to their expertise, their expectations, and the context in which the event arises (e.g., Neisser, 1979;

Norman, 1968), and this same effect undoubtedly also holds true in experimentation. In other words, what experimenters observe depends substantially on their familiarity with the experimental setting, their a priori predictions, the relationship of a particular observation to like observations in related experiments, and their general ontological models of the world and reality.* For precisely this reason two experimenters can observe the same phenomenon and interpret it quite differently. The contrasting interpretations of the observed phenomenon of invariant relative timing given by theorists with opposing views on the control of movement provides a good case in point (e.g., see Kelso, 1986, and Schmidt, 1985). With this in mind we should abandon the notion of intersubjective agreement as an essential element of an experiment and note rather the importance of knowing something about the experimenter's expectations, cognitions, and mental models of the world as a means of understanding more clearly the experimentation process. It should be clear that experimentation is not null and pure; it is an intellectual activity in which individual differences in perception and symbolic cognition form an integral part of the whole process.

When Observation Becomes Experimentation: The Addition of Control

Accurate, intelligent observation alone does not make a particular experience an experiment. Wundt (1907) noted that an experiment is a very special type of observation.

> *Experiment* is observation under the condition of purposive control by the observer of the rise and course of the phenomena observed. *Observation*, in the narrower sense of the term, is the investigation of phenomena without such control, the occurrences being accepted just as they are naturally presented to the observer in the course of experience. (p. 22)

Experimentation, then, differs from ordinary experience in that experimentation uses a plan to expose and scrutinize some specific feature or features of the environment through careful control of key features of the event of interest.

Since the time of Wundt, several different meanings of *control* have evolved within experimentation (Boring, 1954). Basic to each is the elimination or neutralization of sources of influence from the phenomenon to be observed. One meaning of control involves the experimenter's checking or verifying an observed relationship by concurrently examining events that lack key features of the phenomenon. In this context control groups

---

*Indeed, many philosophers of science (e.g., Quine & Ullian, 1970) view belief as a foundation stone of science.

are formed to provide baseline observations on a given phenomenon. In studies of the personality characteristics of athletes, for example, control groups of nonathletes provide the baseline data upon which the specific influence upon personality of sport involvement (or preselection toward sport) is assessed.

A second type of control relates to minimizing extraneous influences upon the variables of interest by restraining or maintaining consistency within the experimental conditions. For example, Fitts (1954) developed a reciprocal tapping task that enabled him to study informational constraints upon movement control by keeping the perceptual and decision-making aspects of the task constant and minimal across all variations in tapping-task complexity.

A third type of control involves purposefully guiding or directing a variable to explicitly alter its relationship with another variable. Experimenters in sport psychology, for instance, frequently examine the effect of anxiety upon performance by deliberately adding to the performance situation stressors that are known to affect performer anxiety.

A final type of control relates to the measurement of covariation of relevant, but nonfocal, variables to directly ascertain relative contributions to the phenomenon. Anthropometric variables such as height and weight, for example, are frequently treated as covariates in studies in which motor development researchers attempt to chronicle the time course of the acquisition of the fundamental motor skills of running, jumping, kicking, and throwing.

A major problem for the experimenter is that the imposition of the experimental control needed to understand a particular phenomenon may interfere with and in some way alter the phenomenon the experimenter is trying to understand. Experimental situations in which intervention significantly changes the phenomenon under study may provide only information that is conceptually sterile. In studying phenomena as complex as those involving human action, the experimenter inevitably faces a trade-off between natural conditions with poor control over the variables of interest versus contrived conditions with good control. The ideal of a representative design (Brunswick, 1952) in which the experimenter is able to maintain the phenomenon of interest (in our case complex human movement) in its natural context yet control all extraneous variables that may confound simple understanding of the cause-effect relationship between relevant variables has proven difficult, if not impossible, to achieve in studies of psychology in general, and in the various branches of human action research in particular.

The historical bias in experimentation in mainstream psychology and in human action research has favored the physics model of reductionism and has emphasized experimental control to the detriment of the maintenance of reality in the experimental setting, or what Neisser (1976) has termed ecological validity. Recent calls for increased applied, field-based research, in which phenomena are studied in their natural settings, have been evident in cognitive (Jenkins, 1974; Neisser, 1976), developmental (Bronfenbrenner, 1977; McCall, 1977), and social (Argyris, 1975; McGuire, 1973) psychology. These studies indicate a strong movement away from the traditional bias toward control. This renewed concern with ecological validity within experimentation is also apparent in motor learning and control (Salmela, 1979; Whiting, 1980, 1982), motor development (Rarick, 1982; J.R. Thomas, 1989) and sport and exercise psychology (Martens, 1979, 1980; Whitson, 1978), and the impact of this trend will be considered in other parts of this book.

Contrasting Views on the Experimentation Process

Having ascertained that directed observation of phenomena under carefully controlled and selected conditions is essential for experimentation, we now move to the next important issue: how an experiment is conceived and how the experiment plays its role in the development of scientific knowledge. An important contrast can be drawn here between conventional views of experimentation and some alternative means by which experimentation works in practice.

The Conventional Theory-Driven View

The ultimate aim of science is to produce theories that (a) provide accurate and economical (parsimonious) accounts of known facts within a field, (b) explain phenomena through the identification of causal links between variables rather than merely describe the phenomena, and (c) produce directly deducible predictions that can be supported by empirical testing. Experimentation provides the vehicle through which theory can be evaluated, but is the relationship between theory and experimentation necessarily a unidirectional one?

The typical view of the experimentation process (e.g., Lachman, 1960) is of a rational, logical process that proceeds through a fairly strict sequence of operations from problem formation all the way to the generation of facts that contribute to knowledge. The following sequence of operations outlined by Bunge (1967, p. 7) is typical of the normal, orderly view of the requirements of scientific research.

1. Ask well-formulated and likely fruitful questions.
2. Devise hypotheses both grounded and testable to answer the questions.
3. Derive logical consequences of the assumptions.
4. Design techniques to test the assumptions.
5. Test the techniques for relevance and reliability.

6. Execute the tests and interpret the results.
7. Evaluate the truth claims of the assumptions and the fidelity of the techniques.
8. Determine the domains in which the assumptions and the techniques hold, and state the new problems raised by the research.

Within this conventional view, the experimentation process is usually depicted as cyclic (see Figure 1.1) to acknowledge that the knowledge generated from one experiment guides the formation of the question and hypotheses for the next. The output of one cycle of the experimentation process, therefore, becomes the input for subsequent experimentation on the same problem. Although experimentation is depicted in this scheme as cyclic, the preexistence of theory is the driving force for experimentation, with the experimentation cycle initiated and driven in a strict top-down manner. The initial formulation of theory exerts an overriding influence on all subsequent decisions that are made concerning experimentation. The initial theoretical premise influences, among other things, the operational hypotheses that are formulated, the type of experimental methodology that is selected, and the manner in which the collected data is analyzed and interpreted.

The textbook view of experimentation as a strictly sequenced top-down process is perpetuated by the standardized form in which experimentation is reported. The conventional form of reporting on completed experimentation implies, through its structural subheadings, a logical progression. The introduction section asks a general question, reviews pertinent literature, and forms testable hypotheses. The methods section explains the

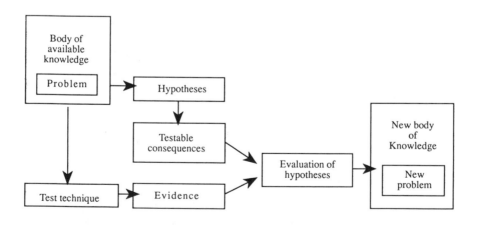

Figure 1.1   A typical view of the research process and the notion of prescriptive stages. From *Scientific Research I: The Search for System*, by M. Bunge, 1967, Berlin: Springer-Verlag, p. 9. Reprinted with permission of M. Bunge and Springer-Verlag.

selection of subjects, apparatus, procedures, and data analysis techniques. Finally, the results and discussion section presents and interprets data, assesses the truth of the original hypothesis, and derives implications of the new data for the body of knowledge.

Such structuring reinforces the dominant beliefs that science is a logical, sequential process and experimentation is the center point of knowledge generation. Examples of theory-driven research within the human action domain are relatively easy to find. Examples include testing the closed-loop and schema theories of Adams (1971) and Schmidt (1975) in motor learning and control, testing neo-Piagetian notions in motor development (e.g., see Thomas, chapter 9 of this volume), and testing theories of achievement motivation and causal attribution in sport psychology (e.g., see Roberts, chapter 12 of this volume).

Although theory-driven experimentation of the type outlined in the conventional view of the scientific process is both possible and indeed desirable (Stelmach, 1987), and the use of a theoretical framework is frequently presented as an important criterion for manuscript acceptance (e.g., see Safrit & Patterson, 1986, Table 3), it is clear that some, indeed most, experimentation does not involve direct theory testing. Landers, Boutcher, and Wang (1986a), for example, in a retrospective inspection of publications in the sport and exercise psychology domain, highlighted how less than 20% of papers within the *Journal of Sport Psychology* involve direct theory testing. These data, and similar data from other areas of experimentation (e.g., Levey & Martin, 1988), show that experimentation need not be theory driven and that rather the research cycle can be initiated from process levels other than theory. In particular, it appears that the experimentation process may also be initiated at the level of data itself and at the level of methodology.*

Alternative Views: Data-Driven and Method-Driven Experimentation

Drawing a distinction reminiscent of those used in models of attention in cognitive psychology (e.g., Norman, 1968, 1969), we can say that experimentation consists of either research that is conceptually driven by a priori theory in a top-down manner or research that is driven by the collected data in a bottom-up manner. When experimentation is performed in a bottom-up manner, theory does not exist in an a priori form but is rather invoked post hoc in an attempt to explain the observed data. New phenomena are typically discovered either as unexpected by-products of other theory-driven research or, more frequently, as conse-quences of an experimenter simply conducting exploratory "look-and-see" experiments in which variables are manipulated and examined but

---

*Note that our definition of an experiment in Part I did not include origin from theory as an essential element.

with no prior rationale (with the possible exception that the experiment has not been done previously) or a priori prediction as to probable outcome. When new phenomena are discovered, the researcher typically proceeds by searching both for replication and for related phenomena, and it may be some time and many experiments later before an explanatory theory is proposed that will support conventional top-down experimentation. In the relatively new human action fields in which there is an enormous range of new phenomena available for discovery, it is not surprising that bottom-up styles of experimentation are common. Experimentation is driven as much from the level of collected data as it is from the level of theory.

Some examples of data-driven or bottom-up experimentation in the human action fields include the following:

• *Motor learning and control:* experiments that examine the relative effectiveness of different practice routines (e.g., varied instructional devices, rest intervals, types of feedback provision, and mental-physical practice combinations) with little a priori theory to guide prediction about which set of practice conditions is most likely to be of greatest benefit to learning and performance

• *Motor development:* the documentation of developmental "ages and stages" on various motor tasks in the absence of preexisting theoretical predictors as to why certain developmental sequences might emerge preferentially

• *Sport and exercise psychology:* identification of the characteristics of successful athletes, teams, and coaches with no preexisting theoretical premises as to what characteristics to expect or how such characteristics develop

A powerful influence on experimentation, which is rarely accorded the recognition it deserves, is the influence of new techniques, equipment, or methods of analysis. A whole class of experimentation can be, and we believe should be, recognized in which the initiating or driving force in the experimentation process is methodology. In method-driven experimentation, the researcher starts with the new technique and then seeks problems to which the technique can be applied. Theory and data then emerge as consequences within the experimentation cycle rather than as prime movers (as the conventional view would have us believe). Method-driven experimentation, not surprisingly, is frequently characterized by a lack of theory, and its principal contribution to knowledge advancement is often limited to providing a more complete description of the assumption and limitations of the particular technique than existed previously. Such contributions are, nevertheless, vital and form an essential step in the integration of new technology into the routine theory-driven and data-driven approaches of the field.

In the human action field, one can readily find examples of the application of new technology in the absence of a priori theory. Increased accessibility of apparatus for kinematic and kinetic analyses of human motion in the mid-1970s and early 1980s, for example, gave rise to a whole class of experimentation both in motor learning and control and in motor development that was, in the early stages at least, devoid of substantial a priori theory. It is only recently that theoretical premises were established (based on nonlinear dissipative dynamics) (e.g., Kelso & Kay, 1987; Kugler, Kelso, & Turvey, 1980; Newell, 1985a) that actually required such methods. Similar instances can be found in sport and exercise psychology with respect to the ready availability of psychophysiological recording equipment. Method-driven experimentation in such cases typically precedes conventional theory-driven experimentation rather than being dependent upon it.

Although it is undoubtedly true that theory development and confirmation are essential for the growth and maturation of any field of scientific study (e.g., see Landers, 1983; Stelmach, 1987), it is equally true that theory development and confirmation comprise a slow, cumulative process. As a consequence, much experimentation occurs in ways other than strict top-down fashion, being frequently driven and initiated in the absence of a priori theoretical notions. Recognizing these alternative approaches to experimentation is important if we are to gain a more realistic view of the experimentation process than is conventionally provided in textbook presentations of the scientific method. As Bachrach (1965) noted, "People don't usually do research the way people who write books about research say that people do research" (p. ix). The experimentation cycle can be initiated at a number of points (see Figure 1.1), and the autobiographical accounts in chapters 2 through 13 will show us that established experimenters often creatively use different types of experimentation (theory-driven, data-driven, and method-driven) in furthering their (and our) understanding of human action.

Stages in the Experimentation Process

Now we consider in some detail the kind of decisions the experimenter is forced to make at each of the stages conventionally involved in the experimentation process. The order in which we consider these steps is roughly in keeping with the usual serial presentation of the experimentation process (as in Figure 1.1), although experimentation does not always proceed in a strict sequence. The autobiographical accounts of eminent researchers in motor learning and control, motor development, and sport and exercise psychology demonstrate that discrete stage conceptualizations of experimentation of the type depicted in Figure 1.1 are often inaccurate representations of the experimentation process in practice. On occasion some of the essential stages in the experimentation process occur simultaneously (e.g., data collection and interpretation; Bartlett, 1958), some retrospectively (e.g., theory-based explanations and rationale for a given experiment often follow rather than precede data collection), and others in orders unique to individual researchers and research projects.* This lack of fixed order creates some problems in interpreting written reports of experimentation, because the structured report may bear little resemblance to the steps and cognitions that accompanied the original experiment. An additional problem associated specifically with simultaneous data collection and interpretation is that the pattern of data return can have a very powerful influence upon how a given set of data is actually interpreted (DeMonbreun & Mahoney, 1976). For these reasons, the division and order of the stages of the experimentation process that follow are somewhat arbitrary.

Selecting a Research Problem

This stage of the experimentation process involves finding an appropriate area within the general field of study in which to attempt to advance knowledge through experimentation. The task of problem selection is driven by a number of factors. The conventional view of experimentation leads one to believe that the selection of a problem area is driven either by a comprehensive review of existing literature that indicates major omissions in the knowledge base of the field or by the desire to tidy up some of the loose ends within the field by performing experiments involving subtle modifications and extensions to existing research studies. Although these kinds of logical selections of research topics do occur, many research problems are arrived at in a more speculative fashion, with researchers deciding to address given problem areas (however narrow) largely because no one has looked at the particular problem or aspect of the problem before. Such data-driven experimentation can be productive when unanticipated but systematic patterns of data are uncovered. However, such a means of selecting a research problem may also hamper the general progress of the field if it allows experimenters to avoid deciding precisely what the right questions are to ask within their particular field of study. Many scientists, including movement scientists (e.g., Connolly, 1970a), regard the problem of asking the most appropriate questions as being at the very heart of knowledge development. The long-term progress of any field clearly requires its experimenters to give careful thought to problem selection.

In addition to being influenced by the experimenter's perception of the existing state of knowledge within the field, the selection of an appropriate

---

*Indeed, in this regard, a serial model of the experimentation process is inappropriate for many of the same reasons that serial stage models of human information-processing have proven inadequate (e.g., J. Miller, 1982, 1983).

problem to study is also strongly influenced by a number of other factors not typically depicted in the textbook version of the scientific method. These include the following:

- Pragmatic concerns, relating to the need to find solutions to practical problems. (In this regard sport and exercise psychology, because of its direct professional link, is arguably more influenced by consumer forces than is either motor learning and control or motor development, although both these fields are increasingly subject to issues of practical accountability; Christina, 1987, 1989; Magill, 1990.)
- The interests and abilities of available colleagues (and supervisors, in the case of graduate students) and the availability of appropriate material resources to support research in the problem area.
- The availability of external grant money to support the research (e.g., Fishman & Neigher, 1982). (The net effect of economic constraints is that externally funded and contracted research must be accountable. The search for tangible outcomes from research grants biases the problem selection of researchers in the direction of applied research.)
- The personal interests, background, and self-perceived capabilities of the researcher.

Many of these external influences (constraints) upon problem selection may, in the short term, turn out to be positive, forcing a field like motor learning and control to increase its attention to applied research problems (cf. Christina, 1987, 1989). However, although applied research has been clearly underrepresented in the history of each of the human action fields, and although all these fields may well benefit from "user" pressures, it should be equally clear that caution needs to be exercised to avoid an unproductive swing in research orientation away from basic research. The history of science shows that basic research (i.e., research that searches for fundamental processes and understanding) consistently leads to more substantive long-term advances in both theoretical and practical knowledge than does outcome-driven research. In considering changes in research orientation by eminent researchers, including those represented in this book, carefully consider whether these changes have been driven by the experimenter's belief that the problems of the original area of enquiry have been fully solved (or have been progressed as far as possible) or whether changes have been driven by the extrinsic constraints imposed upon the experimenter.

Getting Ideas and Forming Hypotheses

Although the actual genesis of ideas is difficult to pinpoint, important ideas and conceptual breakthroughs arise equally often by accident, through a serendipitous finding or a flash of inspiration (the "Eureka, I have it!" sensation), as they do through logical, systematic planning (Cannon, 1940; E.R. Jones, 1988; Mach, 1896). This led Planck (1949) to suggest that the successful experimenter "must have a vivid intuitive imagination, for new ideas are not generated by deduction, but by an artistically creative imagination" (p. 109) and Polanyi (1958, 1967) to argue that tacit knowledge, knowledge based on the integration of personal, experiential insights and intuition, is the essence of scientific creativity. If tacit knowledge of the type outlined by Polanyi plays an important role in the formation of research ideas, then individual differences in background, modes of thinking, and exposure to ideas from beyond the normal bounds of the field of study will greatly affect the type of research ideas different experimenters are likely to generate and apply to the problems of their fields. This theme is developed in greater detail in chapter 14, which considers some of the common characteristics of eminent action researchers. The theme is an important one to keep in mind while reading the autobiographic accounts in chapters 2 through 13.

The extent of individual differences in idea formation may account, in part, for the tendency of experimental work in many branches of science, including psychology (D. Cohen, 1977), to proceed not as one might expect—by building on the foundations of existing experimentation performed by others—but rather by commencing hypothesis formation and enquiry at the level of the original problem. Scientists in general proceed not by adding their bricks of knowledge to the wall of knowledge partially built by others but by starting their own walls (cf. Forscher, 1963). Such a strategy is not as counterproductive as it might appear, and indeed one can argue, as Kuhn (1962) has, that major advances in science depend upon unshackling the constraints of a given line of thinking and returning rather to the level of the original problem. The gains in personality research in sport and exercise psychology, which were made when some of the early trait approaches were abandoned and the associated body of research discarded (e.g., Morgan, 1980; Rushall, 1975c), provide a good example of this point. We next discuss Kuhn's ideas on cycles of science in greater detail.

Selecting an Appropriate Experimental Paradigm and General Methodology

At this stage of the experimentation process, the experimenter must decide what theory-method combination (or experimental paradigm) to use. Once this issue is resolved, the experimenter must make more logistical, but nevertheless important, decisions concerning the level of analysis at which to operate, the type of experimental setting to utilize, and the type of subjects to be tested. If method-driven experimentation is being undertaken, the experimentation cycle may commence with solutions to some of these logistical questions and work back to the more interpretative issues relating to theory selection.

We may best consider paradigm selection within the framework of Kuhn's (1962) historical distinction between *revolutionary* and *normal* science. Kuhn's work is arguably the most important and often-cited single work on the philosophy of science, and the interested reader is directed to the original work (Kuhn, 1962), some updates by Kuhn (Kuhn, 1970, 1973, 1977), plus some philosophical critiques of his work (Bloor, 1971; Chalmers, 1982; Lakatos & Musgrave, 1970). Applications of Kuhn's notions to psychology can be found in Kendler (1981), Mahoney (1976), and Weimer and Palermo (1973), and to the fields of human action research in Martens (1987), Stelmach (1987), and Abernethy and Sparrow (1992).

Kuhn pointed out that the history of science is characterized not by the steady accumulation of knowledge through experimentation, as a linear model of science might predict, but rather by "noncumulative developmental episodes in which an older paradigm is replaced in whole or in part by an incompatible new one" (Kuhn, 1962, p. 91). Kuhn conceived of science progressing through a cycle: pre-science, normal science, crisis and revolution, new normal science, and a new crisis (see Figure 1.2 on page 16). Thus the development of appropriate paradigms of study is characterized by replacement of existing paradigms rather than emergence from existing paradigms.

Normal Science.   Normal science is the activity that occupies most experimentalists' time, resources, and personnel in the scientific field. It is characterized by the steady accumulation of knowledge within a fairly narrow topic area through the use of a widely accepted paradigm. The mass of research conducted in cognitive psychology within the framework of the information-processing model is a good example of prototypic normal science. The principal activity within a phase of normal science is empirical data collection along with attempts to refine accepted theories within the narrow confines provided by the dominant paradigm.

The availability of an accepted paradigm for study inevitably attracts a group of adherents (the "normal scientists"?) in such a collective manner as to be euphemistically labeled the "herd effect" (Landers, 1983). Normal scientists are kept busy by operating on a range of issues arising within the "intellectual structure" (Kendler, 1981, p. 137) created by the dominant paradigm of the time. This research activity is something of a mopping-up operation in which loose ends are tidied up, and the research is characterized by a certain sameness with relatively minor (arguably, trivial) variations of the same basic research logic and experimental method addressed apparently ad infinitum.

Numerous examples of normal science can be found in the literature on human action research. Some of the better examples include research

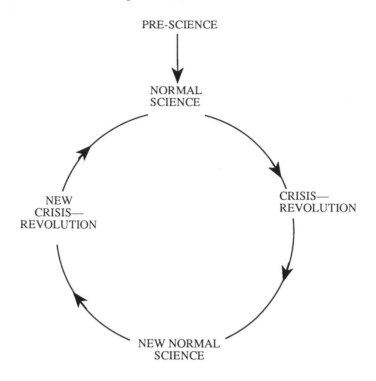

PRE-SCIENCE

NORMAL
SCIENCE

CRISIS—
REVOLUTION

NEW
CRISIS—
REVOLUTION

NEW NORMAL
SCIENCE

Figure 1.2   A schematic view of the stages in knowledge progress in science according to Kuhn (1962).

within the motor learning and control field in which all manner of combinations and permutations of the distance-location paradigm are used to examine motor short-term memory phenomena; research in sport psychology using developed questionnaires such as Martens's (1977) SCAT or Nideffer's (1976b) TAIS with different populations of subjects or different situational conditions; and research in motor development in which age normative changes in the performance capabilities of children are described for as many fundamental motor skills as possible.

Revolutionary Science.   Revolutionary science involves a complete change in focus as a new research paradigm emerges, competes with, and attempts to overthrow the existing one, vying for its own acceptance as normal science. The following sequence of events usually heralds the arrival of revolutionary science and in turn the foundations for a new dominant paradigm of normal science.

During the course of normal science, findings arise that are anomalous to the prevailing theory and paradigm and that the experimenter cannot easily incorporate by modifying the existing theory and paradigm. In response to these findings, the experimenter more extensively investigates the area of anomaly and usually attempts active modifications on the existing paradigm in order to accommodate the new, discrepant data. Supporters of the existing paradigm typically show resistance to change even though the alterations made to the existing theories are usually not completely satisfactory. As Kendler (1981) noted, "the adherents of the existing paradigm learn to live with or, perhaps more properly speaking, to ignore the inconsistent results" (p. 137), and scientists who have developed successful programs of research within the existing paradigm show extreme reluctance to change their viewpoints in the face of the conflicting evidence (Mitroff, 1974a, 1974b). Anomalous results, over the long term, typically inspire researchers, frequently younger and less emotionally attached to the original paradigm than the adherents, to formulate an alternative theoretical explanation for both the anomalous data and the preexisting data supporting the current theoretical position; this ultimately introduces a competing paradigm.

Over time, although the older paradigm is usually retained by those who have worked with it (and grown up with it), the newer paradigm is slowly accepted and adopted, the older paradigm becomes outmoded, and a new order is established with the newer paradigm dominant. The transition between the two paradigms (Kuhn's period of crisis) is an unstable and volatile period, in which emotion as much as logic appears in debates between the proponents of the old and new paradigms. Ultimately, the new paradigm becomes dominant and established, setting in progress another phase of normal science, which continues until a new set of anomalous data emerges and the cycle of revolution is set in progress again.

The current debates in motor learning and control between the established information-processing paradigm of top-down cognitive control and the emerging dynamical, ecological paradigm provide perhaps the best current examples from the human action field of paradigmatic crisis and the enacting of revolutionary science (Abernethy & Sparrow, 1992; Beek & Meijer, 1988). Cycles of normal and revolutionary science are also evident throughout the general history of motor control theories (Abernethy & Sparrow, 1992; Dickinson & Goodman, 1986), although many of the revolutions within the human action field are probably more microrevolutions than major paradigmatic shifts (Martens, 1987).

Understanding the Kuhnian notion of cycles of progress in science is important, as is identification of the dominant paradigm, because the dominant paradigm ultimately determines, in both overt and covert ways, what is normative and acceptable in experimentation. Prime movers in the formation of given paradigms of normal science (and hence "old revolutionaries") inevitably become the gatekeepers (i.e., editors and reviewers) of the major journals and publications in the field and hence, in many respects, gain control over the normal science they have introduced. This in many ways helps to preserve and perpetuate the dominant paradigm, as does the attraction of top graduate students to the designated leaders ("normal" scientists) in the field. With these subtle forces in place to maintain the dominant paradigms, revolutionary science is vital for knowledge advancement and for broadening the horizons of understanding.

Retrospective classifying of landmark research by experts in given fields (e.g., Diamond & Morton, 1978) inevitably reveals that the research deemed to be most critical to a field's advancement is that which changes the method of looking at a given problem and which ushers in with it a large amount of subsequent research activity (i.e., new normal science). This role of revolutionary science in providing new paradigms and new methods of looking at the problems within a given field of study is also well illustrated by Jordan's (1968) comment on the factors that limit knowledge advancement in psychology:

> It is not that facts are lacking; if anything we are overwhelmed with facts, we have far too many facts at our disposal. What seems to be needed are new ways of processing the facts, new ways of *thinking* about the facts. (p. 2)

Choosing Between Normal and Revolutionary Science.   Given the obvious importance of paradigm changes, yet the resistive strength of normal science, the experimenter's task in selecting an appropriate paradigm within which to conduct any given experiment is not simple. The dilemma is whether to operate within the creative restrictions of normal science or to speculate and use a new paradigm that may ultimately prove to be more productive but which, in the short term, may prove both troublesome and difficult with which to gain acceptance. Somewhat paradoxically, established experimenters are best positioned to experiment with novel paradigms, but because of their roles in the development of the normal science of the day, they are also the ones with most invested in the dominant paradigm and therefore the ones least likely to challenge it. A number of examples of normal and revolutionary science are provided in the brief descriptions of the history of and current issues and trends in each of the three fields of human action research that are contained in this book; a number of the autobiographical chapters (e.g., Roberts, chapter 12) also describe the tensions that develop during periods of paradigm crisis.

Selecting an Appropriate Level of Analysis

A problem faced by all experimenters is the selection of a level of analysis appropriate to the phenomenon under observation. This selection problem is especially pronounced in the human action field, where the multidisciplinary nature of the subject matter presents the experimenter with an enormous range of potential observational and analytical tools and levels. As when selecting an appropriate paradigm, the experimenter selecting a single level of analysis must make some kind of compromise.

If the experimenter chooses a micro level of analysis (as a motor control researcher might do in performing a neural-level analysis on single motor unit control, for example), the benefit to be gained is an improved chance of observing and understanding fundamental properties of how the system functions in isolation. The problem with such a fine-grained level of analysis is that one necessarily sacrifices analytical breadth for depth, and the overriding concern becomes the question of representativeness (i.e., how representative is the single isolated system of the whole system). In moving from the use of surface electrodes to monitor the behavior of a given muscle to the use of needle electrodes to monitor the behavior of a single motor unit, for example, one gains increased understanding of the part but to the detriment of understanding the whole. The concern with micro levels of analysis is, therefore, that the obtained observations, although precise for component parts of the phenomenon under examination, may not represent the functioning of all component parts of like structure. Micro-level observations, therefore, may provide only very limited insight as to the interaction of the examined component with other component parts under normal functional operation.

If the experimenter opts for a macro level of analysis, he or she can measure the intact behavior of the whole organism, but underlying mechanisms may remain hidden. As a consequence, an extreme macro-level analysis based, for example, on behavioral observation can typically provide a useful description of a phenomenon but is limited in aiding understanding, in more precise, fine-grained terms, of the underlying functioning of component parts.

Historically experimenters have operated at one level of analysis only, but clearly there are benefits to be gained from the use of multiple levels of analysis. In both motor learning and control and motor development, some of the more exciting recent advances in knowledge have arisen through experiments linking conceptual models of the motor system, derived primarily from behavioral data, with more micro-level data revealed from the use of neurophysiological techniques. Likewise, the combination of behavioral measures of movement outcome with process measures of observable kinematics and underlying electromyographic evidence is proving enlightening. In sport and exercise psychology, studies of individual anxiety responses that have taken concurrent measures at the behavioral, cognitive, and physiological levels have proven more enlightening than analyses restricted to one level alone. Multiple levels of analysis are therefore most appropriately viewed as complementary rather than competing.

The selection of an appropriate level or levels of analysis by an experimenter therefore depends on a number of factors. Foremost among these are (a) the nature of the problem at hand and its receptiveness to micro-versus macro-level examination and (b) the competence and confidence of the experimenter in working at different levels of analysis. The latter is a powerful effect and highlights yet again a potential source of influence upon the experimentation process: the experimenter's unique background, experiences, and personality. In reading the autobiographical accounts of eminent action researchers, note carefully the level or levels of analysis used by different experimenters and consider this within the historical contexts in which their work was performed. In chapter 14 we discuss the use of fixed versus variable levels of analysis by expert experimenters.

Selecting an Experimental Setting

A decision that is frequently coupled to the question of an appropriate level of analysis relates to the setting in which to perform experimentation. The issue here, which was raised earlier in the consideration of experimental control, is whether the researcher should perform experimentation in the natural setting, maintaining all stimuli in their usual context and preserving all the complex interactive effects within the intact skill, or move to a laboratory setting, reducing the research problem to a level that is manageable but artificial. The trade-off, as we noted in Part I, is between the authenticity (ecological validity; Neisser, 1976) of the natural (field) setting and the vigorous control over all extraneous variables that is possible in the contrived laboratory setting.

Psychologists have classically opted for the reductionist methods of the physical sciences, searching for psychological equivalents to the atoms and elements of physics (Kendler, 1981); human action researchers, being heavily influenced by mainstream psychology, have also traditionally opted for laboratory control to the possible detriment of ecological validity (Christina, 1989; Whiting, 1980, 1982). As a consequence the motor learning and control field, in particular, has a dearth of applied field-based research. To a large extent this is a consequence of the predominant view that programmatic research should commence in the laboratory and then move to the field, with progressively more pieces of the intact behavior added as more is understood of the component parts and their interactions. An alternative, more balanced view is that laboratory and field-based research should be viewed as independent but cooperative endeavors (Christina, 1987).

Given the trade-offs, the experimenter's decision whether to perform laboratory or field-based research is a personal, philosophical one. However, whether the experimenter starts in the "real world" setting and then works back to increased control over the variables of interest or starts in the laboratory with the smallest manageable component and attempts to work up to understanding a piece of reality, the overriding concern, we believe, must be that the experiment ultimately contributes in some way to the understanding of real-world phenomena. In reading the autobiographical chapters, look for examples of both laboratory and field-based research and note how a number of the eminent experimenters move between settings in an attempt to gain a more detailed understanding of the phenomena that interest them. The more levels of the laboratory-field continuum an experimenter uses, the better positioned he or she is to discriminate robust and generalizeable effects from level-specific artifacts.

Analyzing Data

Given that the appropriateness of data analysis techniques is one of the key factors in determining whether a manuscript on motor skills will be accepted for publication (e.g., see Safrit & Patterson's 1986 review of the *Research Quarterly for Exercise and Sport*), the successful researcher needs to possess (or at least have access to) expertise in a wide range of data analytic and statistical techniques. Selecting the most appropriate or the most powerful statistical test from the enormous range of tests available, however, may pose a difficult and even daunting task to even the most experienced experimenter. Exponential developments in measurement theory and statistical techniques make it difficult, if not impossible, for the active researcher to keep abreast of these developments in addition to the developments in his or her own area of research specialization.

The drive to keep abreast of both research in the specific field of interest and developments in the measurement and analysis field causes researchers to follow one of three possible strategies with respect to data analysis. Researchers may either secure the services of a professional statistician or else channel sufficient time and energy into the study of analytical methods so as to make the problems of measurement and analysis, in themselves, a focal point of research activity. Method-driven experimentation frequently arises from the latter choice, and a number of examples of method-driven experimentation and of a fascination with measurement and analysis issues are evident in the autobiographies presented later in this book.

As a third means of coping with the complexities of data analytical decisions, many researchers develop competencies in only a limited range of specific analytical procedures and then, with these competencies in mind, design experiments for which these particular analytical tools are suitable. Such a pragmatic approach to analysis allows the researcher to devote his or her time and energy specifically to the research issues of interest. Such an approach, however, carries with it a number of limitations that may, in some instances, brake the advancement of knowledge. For example, univariate statistical procedures (and, in particular, analyses of variance) dominate experimentation in the human action fields (e.g., see Landers et al., 1986a) even though the subject matter of the field is inherently multidimensional and hence more suited to multivariate statistical procedures. Experimenters frequently use multiple univariate analyses where multivariate methods are required (e.g., in the case of multiple dependent measures collected from the same sample) and fail to test the assumptions underlying their routine uses of given inferential tests (Schutz & Gessaroli, 1987). The predominant preference for, and competency in the use of, statistics designed for group-oriented experimental designs also limits understanding of the important contribution that individual differences play in the various human action fields. Because individual differences frequently account for more variance in performance than do many of the independent variables that have been studied in human action experiments (Eysenck, 1966), a strong case seems to exist for the increased use of some of the more recent multivariate methods (e.g., Snyder & Law, 1979) that allow researchers to examine individual differences without the need for single-subject designs.

In reading the autobiographical accounts of eminent human action researchers in chapters 2 through 13, look closely at the kinds of statistical analyses the experts have used, their rationales for selecting these particular approaches, and their flexibility in using different procedures.

Interpreting the Data and Writing the Report

Writing is quite possibly the most important phase in the whole process of science and knowledge advancement. Although experimental design, data collection, and analysis are typically given greater emphasis in traditional texts on experimentation, it is in the writing phase that the actual creating of knowledge occurs. It is on this written form that the value of the research is ultimately judged.

Subjectivity in the Writing Process.   Writing (and hence the presentation of scientific knowledge in its most common yet powerful form) is an abstract reconstructive process, and as a consequence the written form of experimentation often does not directly reflect the development of the ideas for research or the pathway through which the experimental knowledge was actually generated. As Hudson (1972) noted,

> human thought, before it is squeezed into its Sunday best, for purposes of publication, is a nebulous and intuitive affair: in place of logic there brews a stew of hunch and partial insight, half submerged ... although we accept that our minds' products must eventually be judged by the puritan rules of evidence and insight—the straight gate through which they must pass—we seem in practice to draw what inspiration we possess from a hidden stockpile, of images, metaphors and echoes, ancient in origin, but fertile and still growing. (p. 13)

Even Popper (1972), in drawing a distinction between the processes that lead to idea formation and the logical steps involved in testing those ideas (or between what Reichenbach, 1938, termed the *context of discovery* and the *context of justification*), acknowledged that the writing process involves presenting a record of the experimentation process that is not an accurate representation of the actual events in experimentation or of the original cognitions involved in hypothesis formation. Popper (1972) suggested that

> In so far as the scientist critically judges, alters or rejects his own inspiration we may, if we like, regard the methodological analysis undertaken . . . as a kind of "rational reconstruction" of the corresponding thought processes. But this kind of reconstruction would not describe these processes as they actually happen. (p. 31)

The reconstruction process involved with report writing results in, among other things, the recording of fewer and less extensive deviations from the main theme and rationale of the study than typically occur; the process also presents the impression that ideas and experimental testing were developed and performed more rapidly than was actually the case. (Henry, in chapter 2 of this volume, for example, notes that his memory drum concept developed much more slowly than his writings indicate.)

The obvious danger in the writing phase is that the interpretation of the objectively collected data is subject to forces such as personal quirks and prejudices (particularly confirmation bias; Greenwald, Pratkanis, Leippe, & Baumgardner, 1986; Mahoney, 1976); these forces may lead to interpretations beyond what is justifiable within the normal realms of objectivity and rationality. This is particularly true because researchers frequently use inductive inference at this stage of the experimentation process to draw implications from the data that apply to a wider population of events or situations, even though this type of inference does not draw upon the normal rules of logic (Mahoney, 1976). Although processes other than rational logic and objectivity can influence all stages of the experimentation process, the influence of value-laden judgments may be potentially more powerful at this stage than at any other stage.

Constraints in the Writing Process.   Although writing is a creative and potentially value-laden component of the experimentation process, it is nevertheless loosely constrained by the conventional format that experimental reports must follow and by the need to clearly present at least three sound sets of arguments that defend (justify) the experiment's contribution to knowledge. Each set of arguments makes particular claims based on a set of facts, and each one must be related to the next set of arguments so as to produce a new set of facts that can be used in future arguments. The arguments are formed with a similar structure (Toulmin, 1958; Snyder & Abernethy, 1991): the claim to be made, the information or facts upon which to base the claim, and the inference-licenses or warrants that enable the experimenter to draw a particular conclusion from the facts available (see Figure 1.3).

The first argumentative set lays the foundation for the experiment, its importance, and the set of facts from which its hypotheses or conjectures are derived. Usually, the strength of the argument rests on the prior literature about the phenomenon. If the claims appear legitimate, based on the review of "facts," the argument sets the stage for the impending experiment. The claims are the hypotheses that focus the experiment proper, and the set is called the *hypothesis argument*. This is the beginning of the formalities of experimentation. As we saw earlier, experimenters may not actually arrive at their notions based on extravagant deductions from past facts, but once main ideas and particularly hypotheses are formed, experimenters are more than likely to ground their ideas in these formal relationships in order to declare the ideas reasonable for consideration by others. The more extensive the experimenter's knowledge of the area of work, the more likely he or she is to provide new insights. Such is the nature of expertise, when not blinded by overconfidence or complacency.

The second argumentative set establishes the empirical base for the previous assertions. This is the *empirical argument*, and it relates to the adequacy of the experimental design. At this point the experimenter provides arguments to support the claim that the experimental design is good enough to validly expose the phenomenon of interest for scrutiny. In turn, the validity of the findings rests on these claims. If an experiment is adequately designed and planned, the experimenter reaps benefits in terms of weakened counterhypotheses and clearer results. Nature does not often reveal itself easily, so experimenters must use ingenuity and creativity to sort through nature's intricacies.

Experimental findings pose as facts for the last argumentative set, the *interpretive argument*. The claims at this point relate to the theoretical framework. In this way, the planned experience is linked to theory so the experimenter can move from some theoretical orientation, however humble, to empirical evidence, and back to theory. The arguments are the scaffolding for theoretical development. Experimentation serves as counterpoint to the proposed abstractions. Because the arguments are necessarily creative it is often very difficult to map the path between theory and observation, and few experimenters find roads that lead further. The experimenters selected for this book have found some useful paths, ones that may represent the starting points for future work in the movement sciences. Compare the autobiographical accounts in chapters 2 through 13 with the formal reports of the same experiments to see how the argumentative sets become developed in formal writings.

Somewhat paradoxically, leading scientists, especially psychologists (D. Cohen, 1977), report that they enjoy the writing stage of the experimentation process most of all, even though it is the least scientific aspect of their

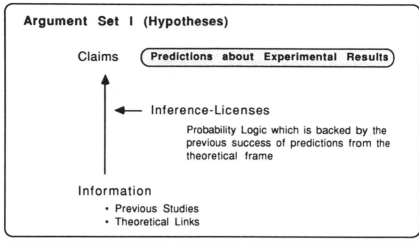

Argument Set I (Hypotheses)

Claims   (Predictions about Experimental Results)

◄── Inference-Licenses

Probability Logic which is backed by the
previous success of predictions from the
theoretical frame

Information
• Previous Studies
• Theoretical Links

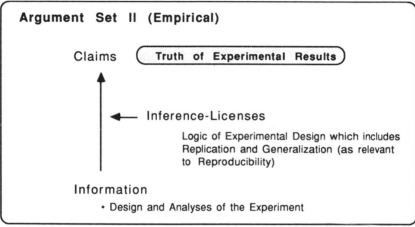

Argument Set II (Empirical)

Claims   (Truth of Experimental Results)

◄── Inference-Licenses

Logic of Experimental Design which includes
Replication and Generalization (as relevant
to Reproducibility)

Information
• Design and Analyses of the Experiment

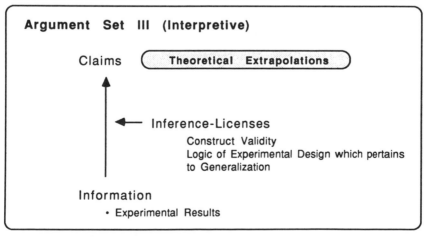

Argument Set III (Interpretive)

Claims   (Theoretical Extrapolations)

◄── Inference-Licenses

Construct Validity
Logic of Experimental Design which pertains
to Generalization

Information
• Experimental Results

Figure 1.3   Experimentation depicted as a set of arguments. From *Experimental Inquiry*, by C.W. Snyder, Jr., & B. Abernethy (1991).

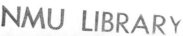

work. Cohen suggests that this occurs because experimenters are most released from the restraining shackles of the scientific method and have most room to create, maneuver, and speculate on their data in the writing phase. The sport psychologist Robert Nideffer expresses such sentiments in chapter 11.

The Publication and Review Process

In order for written work to be published, and hence have an opportunity to become accepted as part of the knowledge base of a field, it must first (for the more widely respected journals, at least) pass through the peer review process. The peer review process represents an interesting and powerful force that reinforces the existing dominant paradigms within each particular area of study and, in Kuhn's (1962) terms, supports the ongoing course of normal science. Experimenters who show competency in using the dominant methods and paradigms of the field (and in many cases those who were at one time responsible for paradigmatic revolution and the initiation of the current stream of normal science) typically come to occupy positions of power on editorial boards of critical journals.* As editors and reviewers, established researchers may act effectively as gatekeepers of the dominant paradigm—a paradigm with which they are most familiar and comfortable and to which they are, in Kuhn's terms, emotionally attached.

Certainly there is evidence from the parent discipline of psychology (see Mahoney, 1976, pp. 92-94) to indicate that the reviewing of manuscripts and the subsequent decisions regarding acceptance or rejection of manuscripts may not always be based on strictly objective and rational criteria (as the traditional view of science would imply). Rather a principal criterion for determining how a manuscript is rated appears to be the congruity between the conclusion reached in the manuscript and the reviewer's own theoretical position on the subject matter. There is little reason to suspect that similar effects do not operate in the movement sciences; certainly the comparable rejection rates for movement science journals (such as the *Journal of Sport Psychology*, 63% rejection in the period 1978-84; Landers et al., 1986a) and mainstream journals (Zuckerman & Merton, 1971) suggest that, in general, researchers in the movement sciences experience similar difficulty in moving their work to the publication stage as do researchers in allied fields.

These hegemonic forces, which reinforce the dominant paradigms within science and reinforce other selective criteria operating at the review/publication process level, create a situation in which the research

---

*A quick perusal of the editorial boards of the main journals in a given field quickly reveals how a disproportionately small number of researchers occupy positions of power on a disproportionately large number of journals.

that appears in the scholarly journals of the field may not truly represent the work in the scientific community in general or, more importantly, indicate the true state of matters within a large body of research. For example, many meta-analyses (e.g., Feltz and Landers's 1983 meta-analytic review on mental rehearsal) reveal different conclusions depending upon whether one focuses upon the published literature alone or also examines the unpublished data. Although many works remain unpublished because of methodological flaws, many publishable, methodologically sound pieces of research are not advanced to the review stage simply because they obtain null or negative results (i.e., either they fail to obtain statistically significant effects or they fail to obtain results consistent with the dominant theoretical perspective of the time).

The fact that such studies do not get published is unfortunate for science and for the progress of the field for a number of reasons. First, anomalous findings are an integral part of the process of scientific revolution and in turn of paradigmatic and knowledge advancement, and to ignore such findings may hold back the progress of the field (Smart, 1964). Second, null or negative findings indicate the "boundary conditions" (Greenwald et al., 1986) under which given theories can and cannot adequately predict data. If nonsupportive data are not published, then these boundary conditions are difficult, if not impossible, to ascertain; as a consequence, theories are typically accorded broader explanatory power than is justified. Finally, the prejudice against null data means that the published research provides an unrepresentative view of the actual balance of experimental evidence on a given topic—a view that is biased toward confirming the existing theoretical position (Greenwald, 1975).

The Experimenter in the Experimentation Process

It is impossible to specify the process of experimentation with a set of hard-and-fast rules and equally unrealistic to portray and teach experimentation skills along these lines (as has traditionally been the approach). Experimentation is clearly a dynamic, not a passive, activity. Bartlett (1958) observed:

> The experimental thinker is in the position of somebody who must use whatever tools may be available for adding to some structure that is not yet finished, and that he himself is certainly not going to complete. Because the materials that he must use have properties of their own, many of which he cannot know until he uses them, and some of which in all likelihood are actually generated in the course of their use, he is in the position of an explorer rather than that of a spectator. (p. 137)

Experimentation may be best viewed as a carefully planned, shared experience between experimenter (observer) and subject that is designed to shed light upon variables of interest to the experimenter (see Snyder & Abernethy, 1991, for further discussion of the conceptualization of experimentation). Such a conceptualization does not deny the importance of rigorous control and objective demonstration of logic in the completed research work (the *context of justification*; Reichenbach, 1938). Nor, more importantly, does such a conceptualization of the experimentation process reduce and restrict experimentation to the level of a prescribed set of sequential stages (as one might gather from reading reports of scientific research). Finally, such a conceptualization does not limit acknowledgment of the fact that many aspects of the experimentation process (such as problem selection and data interpretation) are more creative and artlike than is normally acknowledged.

Understanding Experimentation Requires Knowing About Experimenters

We have seen how the personal attributes, values, cognitions, and philosophies of experimenters may impact the kinds of decisions that are made at all stages of the experimentation process. Knowing something about the experimenter is necessary to understand fully the decisions he or she makes regarding the type of research problem to address, the kind of investigative framework or paradigm to adopt, the level of analysis and setting within which to position experimentation, and the interpretation to place upon the collected data. Although subjective elements play a role in all facets of experimentation (Kendler, 1981, p. 7), the influences of contextual and experiential factors are arguably most pronounced in the interpretative (writing) stage of experimentation.

Interpretation is influenced not only by the pattern of data that arises (DeMonbreun & Mahoney, 1976) but also by the unique way of looking at the world imposed by the dominant mode of thinking of the time and fashioned by the experimenter's own beliefs, educational background, and related experiences. Some good examples of these influences upon data interpretation and theory are available in the field of perception (e.g., Gordon, 1989). The advent of information-processing theories was driven by developments in digital computers, and the emergence of ecological psychology was undoubtedly influenced by environmental concerns. These are prime examples of how the dominant technology and world themes of the day influence theorizing and data interpretation. J.J. Gibson's (e.g., 1961, 1979) direct perception notions exemplify how an experimenter's own unique experiences (in Gibson's case acting as an aviational psychologist) can influence the type of questions that are posed, theories that are formulated, and data interpretations that are advanced. It is therefore clearly essential that all experimenters and potential experimenters be aware of these subjective influences in science in order to better understand the system within which experimentation and "the game of science" (Agnew & Pyke, 1969; McCain & Segal, 1969) operate. Only with such an awareness may we "look forward to an era in which scientific inquiry is seen in the cautiously optimistic light of its fitting role—as a thoroughly human journey rather than some sacrosanct destination" (Mahoney, 1976, p. 175).

A Rationale for the Use of Autobiographical Accounts as a Means of Understanding Experimentation

We have argued in this chapter that typical scientific reports and traditional texts on experimentation and research methods are limited in at least three ways with respect to the insight they can provide regarding experimentation and the pedagogical benefits they provide to young experimenters. Traditional methods texts and scientific reports of original research

- fail to acknowledge the role of creativity in all stages of the experimentation process;
- present experimentation in a serial cookbook manner, although in reality only a portion of experimentation operates in this manner; and
- fail to provide insight into how original ideas, especially ideas that have led to pivotal experiments, originate and how these ideas are developed and modified by the experimenters.

In short, traditional reports on experimentation provide little insight as to the experimenter's decision-making processes throughout all stages of experimentation. In an attempt to cast experimentation in a more realistic (and human) light and to encapsulate more fully the dynamism of experimentation, the next three sections of this book provide first-person accounts of pivotal experiments in motor learning and control (chapters 2 through 5), motor development (chapters 6 through 9), and sport and exercise psychology (chapters 10 through 13). These autobiographical accounts provide insights into the experimenters themselves, their backgrounds, influences on their modes of thinking, and the cognitions that underlie both their research careers and the decisions they make at various points in the experimentation cycle. Although autobiographical accounts are necessarily limited by the accuracy of the experimenters' recall and by their abilities to verbalize the decision-making processes active in their experimentation (e.g., Nisbett & Wilson, 1977), such accounts provide, we believe, an important adjunct to formal written reports of experiments, giving an exposure to experimentation in practice that is lost in the formal reports.

How to Read the Autobiographies

In the sections that follow we have attempted to place the achievements of each expert experimenter within the historical context of the development of each of the human action fields. Separate introductory sections provide necessarily brief introductions to the development and focus of principal issues and trends in motor learning and control, motor development, and sport and exercise psychology. Furthermore, each experimenter's background and unique contributions to his field are also briefly chronicled before each autobiographical chapter in an attempt to ground the experimenter's works in an appropriate context. These details should be of value to those readers who don't have specialist knowledge of the human action fields but who are interested in expertise in experimentation.

In reading the autobiographical chapters, notice how different experimenters became attracted to their research fields, how they formulate their research ideas, and how these formulations are influenced both by the experimenter's background skills and by the experimenter's exposure to influential others. Note how original ideas become modified and refined over time and over successive experiments and how some of the experimenters have induced paradigm shifts and introduced new ways of looking at old problems within their fields. Look also for how the experimenters vary in their use of theory-driven, data-driven, and method-driven experimentation and how each one resolves what type of methodology to use, what level of analysis to adopt, and whether to site experimentation in the laboratory or in the field. By coupling the autobiographies with the formal reports of the same experiments, see how the stages and cognitions involved in many of the pivotal experiments are lost in the formalized reports. Above all look for the enthusiasm and energy the experimenters bring to their work and the strategies they use to deal with frustrations, setbacks, and apparent dead ends. Because the autobiographical chapters vary substantially in their emphases on different facets of the experimentation process, the preface to each chapter provides a guide to important themes and points within each autobiography.

Part II

Autobiographies in Motor Learning and Control

$\mathbf{M}$otor learning and control is that branch of human action research concerned with the processes underlying production, control, and acquisition of motor skills.* The field is broad in its focus, with interests ranging from global basic issues—such as how continuous control of all the nerves and muscles needed in even the simplest movement is achieved by the brain and central nervous system or how movement information is encoded and retrieved as a basis for learning—to specific applied questions—such as how the decision-making skills of elite gamesplayers can be improved or how rapid recovery of normal gait by stroke patients can be best achieved. With such a breadth of focus, the field draws heavily not only on intrinsically developed theories and methods but also from the theories and methods of a number of allied academic disciplines (such as experimental psychology, the neurosciences, physics, and computer science) and a number of related applied fields (especially engineering, rehabilitative medicine, physiotherapy, and physical, speech, and music education). The applied fields provide not only case studies for testing the efficacy of motor learning and control theories and an avenue for the eventual use of such theories but also a source of theory innovation in their own rights.

Historically, the motor learning and control field owes its origins to parallel developments in its two principal disciplinary forebears, experimental psychology and neurophysiology.** Approaches to the behavioral

---

Process, in this context, is used in its broadest possible context to include not only cognitive but also neural and dynamical factors contributing to movement.

**Detailed chronicles of the history of the motor learning and control field are provided by Adams (1987), Schmidt (1988), and Spirduso (1981).

studies of movement have traditionally followed the methods of experimental psychology and have sought to identify at various points in the field's history both the behavioral characteristics and the cognitive mechanisms associated with the learning and performance of motor skills. Over the course of the motor learning and control field's development, the theoretical and experimental emphases have closely matched the dominant paradigms of the day from within the parent disciplines. Early behavioral reports on movement production were based on introspection, and although some of the early works remain influential today (e.g., James's [1890] descriptions of the phenomenon of attention), the interest in movement at this time was only incidental. Movement was used in these early works as a tool for studying cognition, a practice that has continued throughout the modern history of cognitive psychology (Kelso, 1982b). With the advent of scientific psychology in the late 19th century, isolated studies of movement control emerged, the most enduringly influential of which are basic studies on arm movement control by Woodworth (1899, 1903) and the applied studies on skill formation by Bryan and Harter (1897, 1899). After a dearth of motor learning and control research of any type in the first quarter of the 20th century, research work in the 1930s and 1940s was very much task oriented and driven by the need to solve applied motor skills problems. These applied problems arose from practical concerns about personnel selection and training for the flying, vehicle control, and gunnery tasks associated with World War II (e.g., Melton, 1947) and about teaching and coaching in physical education (e.g., McCloy, 1934; Miles, 1931; Tussing, 1940). Craik's (1947, 1948) conceptual insights regarding man-machine similarities and the intermittency of control, combined with Wiener's (1948) information-processing perspective on human behavior and Shannon and Weaver's (1949) mathematics of information processing, irrevocably changed the direction of motor learning and control research, setting in place a computational view of human cognition and action that has dominated not only the motor learning and control field but also experimental psychology for the past 4 decades. In the modern era of information technology and high-speed computing, the notion of the human as a high-speed information-processing device with its own unique hardware and software has proven both appealing and powerful. The information-processing framework has served as the foundation for a plethora of research endeavors aimed at detailing the computational stages in the production of skilled movement and quantifying their associated information-processing capacities and limitations (e.g., Fitts, 1954; Hyman, 1953; Miller, 1956).

Studies in the neurophysiology of movement control have focused much more directly on the biological basis of the motor system, seeking to identify both the structure and function of key receptors and effectors. Studies have particularly focused on identifying and understanding the functional anatomy of the various receptors involved in movement control and isolating essential structures and pathways in the brain and central nervous system through which the neural control of movement proceeds. Early key contributions to the neurophysiology of motor control were made by Sherrington, whose work on reflexes resulted in the generation of the notions of *synaptic transmission, reciprocal innervation, final common pathways,* and *proprioception,* which are fundamental to modern neurophysiology (e.g., Sherrington, 1906, 1940). Key contributions were also made by Russian physiologist Bernstein (1967), whose works, recently popularized by modern "action" theorists (e.g., Greene, 1972; Turvey, 1977; Whiting, 1984), alerted motor learning and control theorists to the importance of considering the physical/biomechanical constraints in movement control along with *functional hierarchies, phase relations,* and *distributed control,* terms that have become part of the language of modern motor learning and control. Improved exploratory and electrophysiological recording techniques in the postwar period have all heightened understanding of the structure and function of all levels of the motor system, although the immense organizational complexity of the brain and central nervous system means that an enormous range of important basic questions still remain unanswered.

Fortunately, the historically distinct streams of behavioral and neurophysiological study have largely converged in the modern era, leaving contemporary motor learning and control as very much a hybrid field of study. Both behavioral and neurophysiological methods of inquiry are now commonly incorporated into single studies or programs of research with the complementarity of the two approaches a key ingredient for the advancement of the field. Neurophysiological knowledge provides the structural architecture upon which the efficacy of conceptual models, arising from behavioral studies, can be realistically assessed.

The modern era of motor learning and control research has been dominated by the information-processing model, with the majority of the major theory developments (e.g., the closed-loop control theory of Adams, 1971; the memory drum and motor programming theories of Henry and Rogers, 1960, and Keele, 1968; and the motor schema theory of Schmidt, 1975) all sharing this orientation. In maintaining close paradigmatic links with mainstream experimental psychology, the motor learning and control field throughout its modern history has emphasized process-oriented, laboratory-based experimentation; movement tasks have been characteristically simple (arguably trivial) ones (such as linear positioning or finger tapping) performed by untrained subjects. The emphasis has clearly been on experimental control and rigor but unfortunately to the detriment of ecological validity. In keeping with stage model premises of information processing (e.g., Sternberg, 1969), studies of perception and action have been typically separated, thus disconnecting the normal perception-action linkages that subjects have learned during their performances of real-world tasks. Simple measures of movement outcome (typically, speed and accuracy scores) have been predominant, and only minimal attention has been paid to the question of how subjects achieve particular levels of performance.

Arising not from the traditional source of cognitive psychology but rather from the theories of modern physics and comparative biology is a contemporary school of thought that challenges not only the orientation of existing experimentation in the motor learning and control field but the very underpinnings of the information-processing model. Proponents of the so-called dynamical or ecological theories of motor control (e.g., Kelso & Schöner, 1988; Kugler, 1986; Kugler, Kelso, & Turvey, 1982; Kugler & Turvey, 1987; Reed, 1982, 1988; Turvey, 1977; Turvey & Carello, 1986, 1988), inspired by the writings of Bernstein (1967) on action systems and Gibson (1966, 1979) on visual perception, have argued that the man-machine metaphor, upon which the information-processing model is built, is inappropriate (see especially Carello, Turvey, Kugler, & Shaw, 1984). These proponents also argue that much, if not all, of the control of movement typically ascribed to centrally represented movement plans or programs may be explicable in generic, material-independent, dynamical terms. This contemporary school of thought highlights the control inherent in the dynamics of muscle itself and in muscle collectives, as well as the informational content of reflected light (and the physical signals for other perceptual systems). Direct links and mutuality between perception and action systems are emphasized, and a research strategy is dictated that searches for the informational invariants that both specify action and provide the basis for unitary control of action. Given the underlying tenet of ecological realism adopted from the writings of Gibson (1979), the emphasis in experimentation is upon the study of natural skills (such as reaching and grasping, catching, and locomoting) performed in real-world settings by trained subjects. This represents a complete break from the historically favored experimental orientations of the field.

For perhaps the first time in its history, the motor learning and control field currently finds itself, in Kuhn's (1962) terms, in a period of paradigmatic crisis. (See Abernethy & Sparrow, 1992, and Beek & Meijer, 1988, for more detailed critique of the current debates from this perspective.) Given the major philosophical differences and orientations underlying the two approaches, the crisis is likely to be a protracted one, and regardless of the ultimate emergence of one view as dominant, the direction of the field is likely to be irrevocably changed. New pressures exist for experimentation on real-world actions, for the consideration of the links between perception and action, for continuous analysis of movement kinematics and dynamics (in addition to traditional measures of movement outcome), and for an enhanced focus on questions related to expertise. Both the information-processing and the dynamical approaches to movement control are now under increasing pressure to address the previously neglected, but practically vital, issues related to learning (e.g., see Magill, 1990; Singer, 1990); for this reason, skill acquisition issues might well be the principal focuses for experimentation in motor learning and control into the 21st century.

The expert experimenters who have contributed autobiographical accounts of experimentation in motor learning and control have all contributed substantially to the development of the modern face of motor learning and control research, albeit from somewhat different theoretical perspectives. Franklin Henry, more than anyone else, was responsible for the development of information-processing models of motor control. His memory drum model (Henry & Rogers, 1960) is the precursor to the modern motor-programming accounts. In contrast, Scott Kelso is one of the prime movers behind the emergence of the dynamical models of movement control through his work on nonlinear limit cycle oscillators (e.g., Kelso et al., 1981) and, more recently, synergetics (e.g., Kelso, Scholz, & Schöner, 1986; Kelso & Schöner, 1987). Robert Singer and John Whiting provide rare examples of motor learning and control experimenters who have retained persistent interest in the issues of learning— Singer primarily from a laboratory-based, information-processing perspective, and Whiting from an applied orientation, initially based on an information-processing perspective but increasingly influenced by the emerging dynamical perspectives. More details on the unique niche and contribution of each of these experimenters to the development of the motor learning and control field, along with important points on their styles and methods of experimentation, are provided in the short introductions that precede each autobiographical chapter.

Chapter 2

Franklin M. Henry

Department of Physical Education
University of California at Berkeley
Berkeley, California, U.S.A.

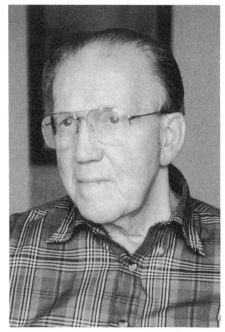

Born in 1904, Franklin Henry completed a BA degree in 1935 and a PhD in 1938 at the University of California, Berkeley. He remains today at this institution as professor emeritus in physical education. Although the field of motor learning and control has historical roots that precede Franklin Henry, arguably no single individual has done more to shape the direction of the field. He is frequently acknowledged as the North American forebear of motor learning and control research (Schmidt, 1988; Spirduso, 1981), and his contributions to the development of the field and also to the general emergence of physical education as a scientific discipline of study are widely recognized and chronicled (e.g., Brooks, 1981; Park, 1981).

Dr. Henry was responsible for the first systematic theory development directed specifically at understanding the control of gross human movement. The memory drum theory of response planning (Henry & Rogers, 1960) posited the view that the control of movement depends on a set of neural commands (a motor program) stored in motor memory and advanced the testable prediction that the time taken to retrieve these commands (as measured by reaction time) directly depends on the task (and hence the control program) complexity. The memory drum concept was based on an analogy to the rotating magnetic drum that was the basic memory device within early electronic computers. The memory drum theory was profoundly influential, and although it has been modified substantially since its original formulation (see Henry, 1981a, 1986, for a more recent version and a review), it provided both the foundation upon which modern motor programming views were based (e.g., Schmidt, 1980) and, perhaps more importantly, the impetus for experimental inquiry and normal science within the motor learning and control field. The memory drum theory represented the first behavioral theory development intrinsic to the motor learning and control field, and it was a timely deviation from the simple adoption of mainstream psychology theories (e.g., those of Thorndike, 1914, or Hull, 1943).

The graduate program established by Henry at Berkeley also provided the breeding ground for a second generation of kinesiology-trained researchers who, from the mid-1960s onward, helped shape not only the motor learning and control field but also the motor development and sport and exercise psychology fields. Prominent human action researchers trained by Henry include Max Howell (now a sports historian), Richard Schmidt, George Stelmach, Ron Marteniuk, and Les Williams (all prominent motor learning and control theorists) and Rick Alderman, Dean Ryan, and Bert Carron (who made their marks in sport and exercise psychology). Through the graduate program, Henry's trademark emphasis on measurement precision, validity, and reliability (e.g., Henry, 1959, 1975) as well as strict adherence to the scientific tenets of control and rigor was spread throughout the United States, to Canada (through Howell, Carron, and Alderman; Wiggins, 1984), and to Australia and New Zealand (via Howell and Williams). Chapter 10, by Bert Carron, provides some insights into Henry's supervision style and influence.

Like many leaders in developing academic disciplines, Franklin Henry also showed a keen interest in professional issues. His most enduring global influence in the physical education field may well be the strong arguments he presented for physical education as an academic discipline in its own right (Henry, 1964, 1978); more locally, his formation in 1966, with Arthur Slater-Hammel, of the North American Society for the Psychology of Sport and Physical Activity (NASPSPA) provided the basis for scholarly interchange between theorists and experimenters in the various fields of human action research. Perhaps less well known to modern students of motor learning and control are the significant contributions Henry made in the exercise physiology field (e.g., Henry & De Moor, 1956; Henry & Trafton, 1951); his knowledge and pioneering research activity in this field ideally positioned him to view the cross-disciplinary potential of the kinesiological sciences.

In this chapter, Franklin Henry describes his early education, the circuitous path that lead him to a career in experimentation in motor learning and control, and some of the cognitions underlying the development of the memory drum theory and related experiments on dynamic kinesthetic perception. In reading Franklin Henry's chapter, note the impact his early experience in electronics had upon his mode of theorizing and upon the analogy he was to select as the basis for his theorizing. Note also how refined theory emerges slowly, even in classical experiments such as those performed by Franklin Henry, and observe how apparently disparate sets of experiments can be drawn together to develop and test global theoretical perspectives. Above all, share in Henry's enthusiasm for experimentation and scientific discovery, and see how this enthusiasm helped him overcome a number of formal educational barriers.

AUTOBIOGRAPHY

My formal education has not been typical. The early years were in city school systems (Seattle and Tacoma, Washington); for grades 6, 7, and 8, I walked nearly 2 miles from our farm in Linn County, Missouri, to a one-room school (white, rather than red). I walked some 3 miles across the fields to my single year of high school in the small town of Purdin, Missouri.

My family consisted of my mother and three boys—I was the middle one. At the age of 14 I decided I could not face a bleak future on the farm (my older brother had already run away from it), so I told my mother that I too was leaving. She agreed to sell the little farm, because her health was failing, but asked how I planned to support myself and prepare for a better future. I replied that I would enlist in the U.S. Navy and attend its aviation mechanics school at North Island (near San Diego), using the false age of 17 years. So I joined the navy. But it turned out that the entrance age for the school had been changed to 18, so I discovered I was an apprentice seaman in the training station at "Goat Island" in San Francisco Bay. Four months later I was a seaman 2nd class aboard the USS *Brooklyn*, the armored cruiser that had been the flagship of Admiral Schley's renowned flying squadron that had acquired fame in the naval battle off Cuba in the war of 1898.

Brooklyn was a coal burner, so every trip at sea was immediately followed by the orders "turn-to all hands, coal ship" and "turn-to all hands, scrub ship." These procedures usually required 2 days. In port, the teakwood main decks were scrubbed down every morning by such as me (that is probably why we were called the deck force) and holystoned weekly. We also conducted landing-party drills, practiced reloading the turret guns, and continuously scrubbed all painted surfaces. This life soon motivated me to study the *Bluejacket's Manual* from cover to cover and qualify for the rating of seaman 1st class, thus becoming eligible for assignment to the electrician's division. (I had learned there was an opening there for a striker, i.e., an apprentice.) By good fortune this transfer was accomplished. Just before *Brooklyn* was placed out of commission in the spring of 1921, I was given the opportunity to take the examination for electrician's mate 3rd class.

So I became a petty officer aboard the USS *Charleston*, where one of my responsibilities was the maintenance of the electrical equipment in the radio room. There I learned the basics of electronic technology. After completing my enlistment I obtained a year of training at the Denver Institute of Technology, a school that had been set up for veterans under the GI bill of the time. I emerged from that year with a government license as radio operator 1st class and a fairly good competence in electronic technology, including radio broadcasting (KOA came on the air in Denver that winter with a powerful transmitter, making it practical for me to build and sell some 50 "crystal" receiving sets).

I then moved to Colorado Springs to be with my mother, and I built, operated, and managed a low-power broadcasting station there. This made it possible for the Colorado Springs Radio Company (which financed my operations) to sell radio sets even during the summer, when static drowned out reception from even the closest large broadcasting stations, located in Kansas City and Denver. Then my mother died, and the economic status of the radio company was not promising.

I had reestablished contact with my older brother; he was just completing his AB at Northeast Missouri State College at Kirksville. He felt that I would be more satisfied with life if I became educated rather than just remaining a skilled, albeit well paid, technician and back-door engineer. This might be my last opportunity to make the shift in personal objectives. Because of my military service, I could enter college at Northeast Missouri State as a special student, not as a degree candidate, and would be on probation until I had proved I could maintain at least a C average. I could take any course I desired if I could persuade the professor to admit me; I could probably support myself as a part-time electrician in the town's electric store.

Because my desire for an education had become both deep and strong, I enrolled at Kirksville. There I completed over 60 semester units distributed among mathematics, chemistry, English literature, art, drama, and of course elementary composition and rhetoric. My grade-point average was well above the required C. By special arrangement I attended courses in bacteriology and physiological chemistry at the Kirksville College of Osteopathy. (These courses were not offered at the state college, but that did not bother me; I was becoming educated!)

One of the trustees of the College of Osteopathy owned a business that manufactured special adjustable tables for surgeons and osteopaths, as well as electrotherapeutic equipment. The diathermy instrument, widely used by physicians and osteopaths in those days for the purpose of applying heat to joints and muscles, was a source of radio interference. This was because its radio frequency currents consisted of high-decrement impulses generated by spark gap excitation of a tuned circuit, consequently creating interferences in every broadcasting receiver within a mile or two's radius. This constituted illegal radio wave transmission. Clearly, federal authorities would shortly take enforcement action to end that problem. I had become acquainted with Trustee McManus when I gained permission to attend courses at the osteopathic college; he had become aware of my radio and electronics background and asked if I could design and test a noninterfering diathermy apparatus. I responded with the confidence of youth and developed a 200-megacycle continuous-wave generator of sharply tuned noncommunication microwaves (a suitable thermionic triode power tube had become available).

McManus put me on his payroll part-time. A year later the job became full-time in his San Francisco electronic medicine research unit; my task was to improve equipment and develop new applications. This transfer meant, of course, at least temporary withdrawal from college. Although I had no college degree, McManus was able to make special arrangements for me to do some research on possible cancer treatments at The Carnegie Institution Desert Laboratory in Tucson, Arizona, which had some unique micrometabolic facilities. When I was about halfway through the project, the Great Depression of the 1930s struck; I was placed on furlough for a year.

Still having a strong desire to obtain an education (perhaps accentuated by my experiences at Tucson), I secured entrance as a special student at the University of California at Berkeley, counting on my savings to finance at least a year of study. My intentions were to enroll in a variety of university courses and also to experiment with the detecting of differences in certain types of sounds, which were of interest to physicians diagnosing diseases of the lungs and abdominal organs by the method of percussion. This would be preliminary to designing a diagnostic electronic device that perhaps the firm could manufacture.

Unfortunately the depression continued and I ran out of money. However, I soon discovered that my talents in electronics and instrument construction were salable on a part-time basis for instrumentation of several research projects in physiology and psychology. I went to the physics department at the University of California, where I hoped to gain the use of a soundproof room. The department chairman thought my problem was interesting but informed me that the soundproof rooms were in the new life sciences building and under the jurisdiction of the Department of Psychology. Furthermore, I seemed already to have the needed background in physics through self-directed extensive reading and practical experience; the psychologists could be of much more help to me because they were knowledgeable about the methodology of measuring sensory capabilities and the testing of human subjects. This seemed odd to me; my theoretical background knowledge of hearing was limited to published studies by the telephone scientists at Bell Labs. I talked with the chairman of the psychology department and found I was welcome. I would be able to use the department's facilities including the apparatus shop, with the understanding that the department could provide no monetary support. Because I planned to make my own apparatus and provide my own materials, that would not be a limitation.

So I became a special student at the University of California, head-quartered in the Department of Psychology but with no expectation of ever receiving a degree. But I had not come to the university to get a degree. At the suggestion of the department chairman I enrolled in two graduate courses: the general seminar (where I would present my tentative problem for critical discussion) and several units of graduate research (because I would be constructing my apparatus and performing experiments). Additionally I enrolled in an elementary course in psychology because I had no real knowledge about that subject. I also enrolled in classes in analytic geometry and one of the upper division breadth requirements.

Thus began my destiny at the University of California in January 1932—I write this in my office-laboratory as professor emeritus of physical education, University of California at Berkeley, in June 1987. Of course much happened between these two dates.

The depression continued; I was able to support myself by redesigning and building apparatuses for faculty research projects in various departments. Later I did routine testing of subjects as an hourly employee for some of these projects. My time commitments were sufficiently flexible that I could continue a nearly normal load in upper division courses that I felt would be important to my education; I made some progress with my own project. Soon I found that I had completed the required courses in the psychology major (with formal emphasis on the experimental and physiological areas) as well as most of the college breadth requirements. I developed several other ideas about needed research as I continued the graduate seminars. Some of these ideas led to experimentation; several of the studies became completed and published papers.

In 1934 I assessed my balance sheet of accumulated course credits and discovered that if I transferred the 60 units from Northeast Missouri State to matriculation credit in order to make up for the 3 years of high school that I had missed, the remaining units would convert me to regular status as a university senior. Following 1 year at a somewhat more than full-time academic load, I completed the BA degree in 1935; I had accomplished the impossible dream. This would have been impossible if the psychology department at the University of California had not encouraged me and opened its facilities to my unorthodox use, or if the university administration had not been reasonably flexible.

The next step was to enter the doctoral program in experimental and physiological psychology at the University of California. An appointment as a teaching assistant also came my way the fall semester in the Department of Psychology and the spring semester in the Department of Physical Education. In the latter department I was responsible for the laboratory sections of the upper division course in exercise physiology and physiological hygiene. Both fall and spring of the next 2 years involved employment in the physical education department only and included considerable responsibility in its MA program under the direction of its chairman-professor. This gave me valuable experience in teaching at both upper division and graduate levels, and it provided a steady source of income for 3 glorious years as a PhD candidate in my area of psychology. Of course there was no time for summer or weekend vacations, but I did not miss that because I was fully involved in the pursuit of knowledge and enjoying life to the hilt; moreover an end result was in sight. I reached it at the close of the summer session of 1938, when I received the PhD degree.

The Department of Physical Education was developing an academic degree program in the liberal arts college; the department made me an offer that emphasized ample time for research and didn't restrict its direction and an opportunity to develop a new academic course in my area of psychology as an aspect of physical education. I accepted the offer in the summer of 1938 in preference to an invitation to teach several courses in lower division elementary psychology in a small liberal arts college with no research opportunities. I have not regretted that decision.

So I became an instructor at the University of California in 1938 and advanced through the various steps to become full professor in 1952. From 1944 to 1957 I held an additional appointment as research associate in the university's Donner Laboratory of Medical Physics, concerned chiefly with the area of aviator's decompression sickness (this was before the days of pressurized cabin aircraft).

The editors have asked me to comment on how I became interested in a particular research topic, developed a scientific hypothesis, and formulated a method for securing factual data to test it. Because the behavior of humans is usually characterized by individual differences as well as considerable variability within individuals (even when observational and instrumental errors are minimal), it is often difficult to decide what evidence needs to be secured in order to lead to general acceptance of some particular theoretical explanation (i.e., develop an understanding of the behavior in fundamental terms). Moreover, most theories that attempt to explain even a relatively limited aspect of behavior such as motor learning and its concomitant memory trace are likely to have multiple aspects, so it should not be surprising that it may be difficult or impossible to identify a particular occasion when the initial concept occurred that led to a theory such as the memory drum theory (Henry & Rogers, 1960).

The term *memory drum* requires explanation. In those days computers used rotating magnetic drum memory, which somewhat later was replaced by the multiple-disk magnetic trace memory. Probably the concept of the theory began with my realization of the implications of the extreme task specificity of even simple learned motor skills (Henry, 1955, 1961). But I was also involved at that time in several experimental studies in the area of exercise physiology and had undertaken a study on dynamic kinesthetic perception as well (Henry, 1953). In any case, it was nearly 1960 before I came to the working hypothesis that the neural organization required in a simple reaction time (RT) experiment involved two independent processes, one concerned with the RT per se and the other with the subsequent movement time (MT), which could be considered as a measure of muscle effectiveness.

Both were actually consecutive phases of a single process; because there was by definition no observable movement during RT latency, individual differences in the movement phase should be correlationally independent of those in the RT phase. Further consideration of this independence phenomenon, along with my personal experiences in learning and using the Morse code while I was a radio operator, also played a part in my development of the memory drum concept (Henry, 1981a). Then it occurred to me that if the movement (performed at maximal speed) that followed the RT was made more complex, the latency period (i.e., the RT) should be longer because it would require more time for the organized outflow of the more complicated motor control program (which would have increased control elements).

I set up an experiment that used three movements. Movement A was a simple finger lift such as those commonly used in RT experiments, the movement being very short and simple. Movement C began as a finger lift like Movement A; the subject then raised the arm to backhand a tennis ball hanging on a string to the right, moved the arm downward to press a button on the baseboard, and then moved the arm upward to grab another ball hanging on a string. The string holding this ball was tied to a piece of metal at its end, which was held by a spring clip, thus completing the timer circuits. When this ball was grabbed the MT timer stopped. Movement B only used the last tennis ball and was thus of intermediate complexity.

I performed the experiment on a sample of 30 college men and another of 30 college women; my assistant, Don Rogers, obtained data on somewhat smaller samples ($n = 20$) of 8-, 12-, and 24-year-olds and subsequently retested them. In each of these five samples the RTs were substantially and significantly larger for B than A, and for C than B. Having this clear evidence in hand, I published an account of the experiment and my thoughts about the working hypothesis of the memory drum theory (Henry & Rogers, 1960). Others, using modified tasks and methods, have obtained supporting evidence (Henry, 1981a, p. 307ff.).

In 1952 or thereabouts I also became interested in kinesthetic perception. While reorganizing the lectures for my course entitled Psychological Bases of Physical Activity, which I had started in 1942, I consulted the various handbooks of experimental psychology as well as the original literature but found little of value to me. I had come to the opinion that an individual performing a motor act in a skillful manner has almost no conscious awareness of the reception of and response to the kinesthetic information essential to the neuromotor control of the muscle action that implemented the act.

So I devised an experiment (Henry, 1953) that would produce some meaningful factual information. First I had to create a situation that would produce a lot of kinesthesia—for example, a shoving match between two individuals. I could replace one of the persons with a shoving machine. This would standardize the shoving and simplify and improve the recording of who did what and what was the response. The machine shoved with a vertical lever about 90 cm (36 in.) long, pivoted 45 cm (18 in.) below the upper end. On that end was attached a square wooden block 5×5 cm (2×2 in.), which served as a handhold (pad) at approximately shoulder height. The human adversary stood in front of the lever, arm flexed at the elbow and with the right hand on the pad; the hand pushed forward, while a heavy spring inside the machine applied a counterforce. This force was continually but irregularly varied between 6.22 and 12.0×10^6 dyn (14 and 27 lb), being controlled by a motor-driven cam of appropriate shape. The position of the lever was continuously recorded automatically by a pen marking on a moving paper tape. A single trial (one cam revolution) lasted 60 s.

There were two tasks. In the first, the blindfolded subject was required to maintain the lever position unchanged, yielding or applying more counterforce as necessary to maintain this constant lever position while the cam varied the force exerted by the apparatus. In the second task, elbow flexion and appropriate muscle adjustments were increased or decreased, altering the lever position as necessary in order to maintain a constant force (pressure) against the hand pad while the cam altered the applied force. Whenever the subject consciously perceived that the pressure was increasing, he or she made a mark on the tape by striking with the other hand a stretched signal cord once; when the pressure was perceived as decreasing, the subject struck the cord twice.

With the lever position constant, maintained by the subject's pushing harder or easing up when the machine pushed harder or eased up, the subject responded accurately but without conscious awareness to a variation of only 0.29×10^5 dyn (0.065 lb; this corresponds to an average

Weber ratio of 0.0032), indicating an extremely sensitive muscle adjustment mechanism.

In the case of the constant pressure task, the results were of a different order of magnitude; the subject responded to a change in applied force of 3.16×10^5 dyn (0.71 lb) by pushing harder or easing up so as to prevent differences in pressure between the subject and the machine as the machine changed its exerted force. In contrast, a change of 5.56×10^5 dyn (1.25 lb) was required if the subject was to consciously perceive change.

Stated as Weber ratios, these values become 0.035 for the adjustment and 0.061 for the perception. Note that the ratio for deep pressure perception is 0.013, suggesting that this type of perception may also have been involved in the constant pressure task, whereas the ratio for cutaneous pressure is 0.136 (Woodworth, 1938), which is so high that it can probably be excluded. Evidently the hypothesis of nonconscious adjustment was confirmed.

This dynamic kinesthetic perception and adjustment study was relatively discrete, was intended to produce some useful basic information, and might ultimately play a part in resolving some important theoretical issues. I suppose it is typical of my research style (if I have one). The memory drum investigation does not fit into that pattern very clearly. Its origin was rather diffuse; the concept very likely developed more slowly even than my writings indicate. The 1960 formulation, in retrospect, was rather tentative; it needed other and definitely different types of supporting evidence, but I had difficulty in determining what they might be, and I needed to incorporate the learning phase explicitly.

My last publication about the memory drum theory was Henry (1986); I believed it to be considerably improved, but I really do not know where or how many of the new insights developed. Isaac Newton, when complimented on his achievements, responded that he stood on the shoulders of giants. Probably much scientific progress comes in that manner, but I believe that more occurs when we stand on the shoulders of less gigantic, and often (although perhaps unintentionally) unacknowledged, contributors to knowledge. The reader who is concerned about the topics addressed in this paragraph may find my 1981 article of interest.

With the Henry (1981b) paper, I attempted to move the memory drum study forward by constructing a numerical model. A set of n random numbers in normal distribution (Clark, 1966) was adjusted by a suitable constant multiplier and additive constant to $M = 14$, $SD = 3$ in order to approximate and facilitate later comparison with real data—this represented the postlearning performance series as determined by the motor memory traces in the n individuals. Next, n sets, each consisting of k random numbers (the e series), were drawn from a random numbers population $M = 0$, $SD = 1$; all members of a particular set had added to them a particular one of the numbers from the $M = 14$, $SD = 3$ set. This created "individual differences" among the n sets of k trials each and trial-by-trial variation in the consecutive scores of each individual. Because that variation would be ephemeral (noncumulative), it would determine the mean level of correlation, but the matrix of r's would exhibit no remoteness effect. This constituted the first type of model.

The second type of model required adding on another k sets of random numbers of $M = 0$, $SD = 0.34$. The consecutive numerals within each set were cumulated (viz., $1c = 1$, $2c = 1 + 2$, $3c = 1 + 2 + 3$, and so on) for the other trials. A correlation matrix calculated from this model was expected to exhibit the remoteness effect; the correlation between adjacent trials (e.g., 1 vs. 2 or 2 vs. 3 or 3 vs. 4 and so on) would be largest. The mean r for each diagonal of the matrix should progressively decrease with more trials interpolated between those being correlated (Trial 1 vs. 3, 2 vs. 4, and so on; 1 vs. 4, 2 vs. 5, and so on). The mean adjacent trial correlation was intended to be about $r = 0.87$ (adjustable by varying SDe). The remoteness effect (adjustable by altering SDc) was intended to drop to approximately $r = 0.78$ between Trials 1 and 20. The values actually produced were $r = 0.90$ for the adjacent trials and 0.83 for the 1 versus 20.

In my 1980 article I presented a graph giving the results with the second model compared with the last 20 trials of postlearning data from the $n = 51$ subjects in the Norrie (1967) speed of arm movement task. Some additional statistics were also calculated: the *covariance* (the variance component representing the memory trace established by the learning period) and the *within-variance*, which included both the ephemeral random error component and the smaller but cumulated random component that alters the memory trace. For technical reasons the r's were converted to z values and the variances were converted to their square roots. (If you look at the graph, keep these conversions in mind.) The slopes of the regression lines of r on the number of interpolated trials evaluate the strength of the remoteness effect; these slopes are remarkably similar to those posited by the model. I interpret this result as confirming the validity of the model as accounting for the cause of the remoteness effect in the real data. Although there is a noticeable vertical separation between the lines for the model and the arm data, that is not important—a more accurate adjustment of the parameters of the model would eliminate that difference.

Obviously the next step was to provide for the learning situation. Soon after the 1981 publication I did this and proceeded to formalize my theoretical ideas about the motor learning and control program. I thought that the program first required some sort of mental "reference image" of the intended action; it would probably involve kinesthetic elements somehow produced by the mental visualization to begin with. Neural output from the image would feed into an "executive," which would recruit preexisting appropriate neural subroutines and form them into a "program proper," which would be stored, and also would result in efferent impulses to the muscles and result in performance. Afferent neural information would then feed into a comparator section of the system, where the reference image was also available, and the discrepancy between program and intended act would be determined. This information would then feed back into the executive and be stored as modification of the program proper. The discrepancy was considered to have two components. The first was a cumulated portion having a positive (i.e., improvement) trend during learning that was stored as part of the revised program proper; the second was ephemeral and vanished after each trial because it was not cumulated on the stored program.

With the theory presented as a block diagram, these concepts can form the basis of a computer analog derived from a numerical model based on the 1981 version modified to incorporate the learning factor. I set up a more extensive model than in the earlier study. It consisted of 50 artificial subjects each performing 24 learning trials. They were processed through the computer, first with the Type 1 model (ephemeral discrepancies only) and then with the Type 2 model that included both ephemeral and the cumulated (stored in memory) discrepancies (Henry, 1986).

Before comparing the complete Norrie data with the newest model, I first looked at the performance trends of each of her 51 subjects. Sixteen of them failed to exhibit significant learning in their 50 practice trials, whereas the other 35 definitely showed learning. The two groups were analyzed separately. Put to the test, the "remoteness" hypotheses derived from the theory were confirmed. The correlation matrices of the learners exhibited a definite remoteness effect in the practice period as well as in the postlearning period. In contrast the matrices for the nonlearners failed to exhibit remoteness in either period.

With respect to the reference image, Morford (1966) performed an experiment using the Henry (1953) apparatus modified to give variable but controlled visual information to supplement that from kinesthetic stimuli. In the absence of the visual supplement, practice failed to produce evidence of learning. When only the largest 17% of maladjustments were visually displayed during their occurrence, the practice resulted in substantial and significant learning when subjects were tested under purely kinesthetic conditions. I interpreted these results as supporting the hypotheses of the reference image in my theory. It is interesting that this specific need for evidence supporting that idea was not yet apparent in 1966. There was also a speculative possibility that the auditory stimuli from the Norrie timing apparatus could have furnished some useful information for the reference image; the Weber ratio for the temporal duration being 0.20 (Henry, 1948) was not small enough to make this idea acceptable.

This 1986 theory of how the motor control program is developed in the central nervous system can be no more than a step along the way toward understanding motor learning and the memory trace. I realize that in my published papers, I have not commented on other and very different theoretical approaches. Do not interpret this to imply that in my opinion they do not represent important contributions to knowledge. Granted, I am limited in my scientific insight, but I am not *that* stupid.

ACKNOWLEDGMENT

I truly appreciate the encouragement and constructive criticisms of Rheem F. Jarrett throughout the writing of this chapter.

Chapter 3

J.A. Scott Kelso

Center for Complex Systems
Florida Atlantic University
Boca Raton, Florida, U.S.A.

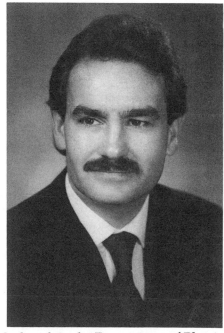

Scott Kelso was born in London-
derry, Northern Ireland, in 1947
and completed his early education
at Stranmillis College in Belfast.
He taught mathematics and English as well as coached rugby and
cricket at Coleraine Academical
Institution in Northern Ireland for
2 years before emigrating to North
America to further his education.
He first completed a bachelor of
science degree at the University
of Calgary, receiving his undergraduate tuition in motor learning
and control from Dr. Barry Kerr.
This was followed with MSc and
PhD degrees from the University
of Wisconsin at Madison in 1973
and 1975, respectively, under the
principal supervision of Dr. George Stelmach in the Department of Physical Education. Kelso also gained valuable research experience at this
time with Dr. William Wanamaker in the Department of Neurology and
Dr. William Epstein in the Department of Psychology, associations that led
to publications on the nerve compression block used to create functional
deafferentation (e.g., Kelso, Stelmach, & Wanamaker, 1974) and attentional
allocation during visual displacement (e.g., Kelso, Cook, Olson, & Epstein,
1975). After a 2-year assistant professorship at the University of Iowa,

Dr. Kelso moved to Connecticut in 1978 to take up a concurrent research appointment at Haskins Laboratories, New Haven, and at the University of Connecticut, Storrs. He remained in those positions until 1986, when he assumed his current post as the Glenwood and Martha Creech Chair in Science and director of the Center for Complex Systems at Florida Atlantic University, Boca Raton. He also holds professorships in the departments of Psychology and Biology at FAU. Scott Kelso is a past editor of the *Journal of Motor Behavior* and a current editorial board member and ad hoc reviewer for a number of influential mainstream and movement science journals.

Like Franklin Henry, Scott Kelso has had an enormous impact on the motor learning and control field, although his contemporary perspective is very much in contrast to the information-processing and motor-programming viewpoint presented by Henry. Kelso's early research work, arising largely from his doctoral dissertation, was very much in the classical information-processing mold, focusing on questions related to motor short-term memory (e.g., Stelmach & Kelso, 1973, 1975) and movement planning (e.g., Kelso, 1977b); however, his influential 1977 *Journal of Experimental Psychology: Human Perception and Performance* paper (Kelso, 1977a) on equifinality and the mass-spring model indicated a transition in interest toward dynamic processes. This transition in focus was accelerated by Kelso's move to Connecticut; exposure to the thinking of Michael Turvey, Peter Kugler, Elliot Saltzman, and others resulted in the formulation of what was, at the time, a radical approach to movement control. The dynamical approach that emerged from these collaborations emphasized the physics of nonlinear dissipative systems as the basic explanatory tool for movement control (e.g., Kelso, Holt, Kugler, & Turvey, 1980), casting the questions posed by movement coordination and control into a whole new perspective and requiring a complete shift in investigative strategy and paradigm. Kelso's conceptual and experimental work on nonlinear limit cycle oscillators (e.g., Kelso, Holt, Rubin, & Kugler, 1981), particularly in terms of temporal entrainment in interlimb movements (e.g., Kelso et al., 1981; Kelso, Southard, & Goodman, 1979) and speech movements (e.g., Kelso & Tuller, 1984; Tuller, Kelso, & Harris, 1983), has been extremely influential in promoting a new line of inquiry into movement control. His recent work on synergetics, especially on phase transitions in coordinated hand movements (e.g., Kelso, 1984; Kelso, Scholz, & Schöner, 1986; Kelso & Schöner, 1987), has provided a vital methodological window not only into the dynamics of control but also, potentially, into the dynamics of learning. Support for the dynamical perspective has escalated in recent years to the point where the popularity of the dynamical approaches now challenges that of the traditionally dominant information-processing perspectives (e.g., Meijer & Roth, 1988), and this is due in no small part to the dynamic presentation of the emergent perspective by Kelso. Kelso's influence has extended beyond the normal boundaries of the motor learning and control field, with his introduction of the dynamical perspective to the problems posed by motor development (e.g., Kelso & Clark, 1982; Thelen, Skala, & Kelso, 1987) and movement disorders (e.g., Davis & Kelso, 1982) also changing the orientation of experimentation within those fields.

In this chapter Scott Kelso elaborates on the thinking underlying the dynamical approach and highlights points of contrast (and advantages as a method of inquiry) between the dynamical approach and the more traditional (information-processing) approach. He highlights essential contrasts between a priori and a posteriori explanations of movement phenomena and outlines the type of investigative paradigm that a dynamical approach to motor learning and control requires. In addition, Scott Kelso's descriptions of his recent work in synergetics provides us with a valuable insight into the questions of creativity in science, especially in terms of how serendipity and intuition frequently impact the development of a research program. His autobiographic chapter also provides a wonderful example of the important role that contact with the modes of thinking of scientists from other disciplines plays in the advancement of theory in a particular field.

AUTOBIOGRAPHY

I take this opportunity to raise a basic question for movement science: What do we mean by *understanding* in the context of animal (including human) action? What language (concepts, tools) and what strategies might facilitate understanding? Here, I wish to advocate an operational approach to understanding movement behavior, in which theory is formulated for observable variables only, and all consequences of a theoretical formulation are checked experimentally. That is, predictions are made that can be experimentally tested. Such a position may seem no more than a restatement of the normal canons of science. But in my view, the gap between theory and experiment in the motor behavior field is far too large, and as a result, a kind of pseudoscience predominates. I do not wish these views to be interpreted as a return to behaviorism: far from it. A science of behavior, on the other hand, rests on the choice of appropriate observables. Movement science, supported by new technologies, provides a much richer set of methodological tools and observables than ever conceived of by the behaviorists (or even by motor behavior research when I first became involved). At present, however, movement science lacks a conceptual framework and an unambiguous language with which to exploit these tools. The first part of this essay addresses the dominant paradigm for explanation in science and attempts to expose some of its weaknesses. In a necessarily cryptic fashion, because of space limitations, I propose an alternative in the second part. In the third part, following the request of the editors, I relate something about how my views have evolved and some of the people and events that influenced them. A short note on the topic of creativity (or the creative juices) closes the essay.

Toward a New Kind of Reductionism

When a scientist is faced with a complex phenomenon like human movement, an orthodox scientific strategy is to decompose the system into elementary units and study their properties. The knowledge gained about such units may be enough for the scientist to understand the behavior of the whole system. This strategy follows a so-called Newtonian world view: Every material system, in principle, can be decomposed into a population of structureless particles moving in fields of force. Dynamical equations governing such populations can be written down and solved. Among many other ramifications and implications, this revolutionary world view has become the canonical form of scientific explanation (see Rosen, 1985).

Take the popular idea of a motor program, strongly advocated by my friend and colleague Richard Schmidt and used frequently as an explanatory construct in both the behavioral and neurological sciences. Although no one has made the linkage explicit (i.e., explained how the contents of a motor program are derived from its neuronal underpinnings), the neural basis of the motor program is assumed to lie in the central pattern generator (CPG), a circuit of identified neurons connected together that generates a motor output. Quite recently, a list of requirements for understanding a CPG has been provided (Selverston, 1980). The list includes identification of all the cells involved, information about all unit properties, and complete knowledge of neuronal connectivity and of all synaptic properties. The list is extremely long, and more than 50 different parameters are involved. If full understanding can only be accomplished this way, there is obviously no need for theory. Theoretical understanding always involves simplification and, by necessity, incomplete knowledge. But if every material detail about a phenomenon is known and incorporated into a model, the end result is a model of everything. A model of everything, however, is a model of nothing. It neither simplifies (because it is so complicated) nor unifies, in the sense that it illuminates principles of organization (e.g., how a pattern is assembled from interactions among subsystems).

Parenthetically, it is interesting to note that neuroscience is now recognizing that the materialist reductionist program, though it has enormously advanced knowledge of cellular and synaptic phenomena, has revealed few insights into general organizational principles of neural and behavioral function. Some have even remarked that the more we discover about the details of each individual nervous system (e.g., in snails, lobsters, or cockroaches), the further we remove ourselves from possible principles. The problem, I think, lies in our failure to abstract essential features of complex systems, combined with a much too narrow focus on matter itself. Let me elaborate briefly.

Insofar as we as biological systems are material systems, the materialist reductionist program is what I call "it" or "thing" based. Fragmentation and decomposition are always into some *thing*, and that something is assumed to hold the key to understanding. The CPG as a fundamental neuronal unit (underlying behavior) is said to contain or represent the actual pattern observed in the real world. The question of how a pattern is formed and generated is thus solved by studying a material object, the pattern generator. The dynamical processes of pattern generation (e.g., stability, flexibility, adaptability, and multifunctionality) are often ignored. This error is analogous to the ancient Greeks ascribing thunder to the anger of Zeus: The modern tendency is to ascribe the processes of pattern formation and generation to a material object located inside the nervous system.

Challenging a dominant epistemological view may seem like a challenge to science itself, although this is obviously not my intent. I want to intimate, however, that a different kind of reductionism is possible: one that fully recognizes not only the system complexity of living things (e.g., in terms of the large number of degrees of freedom involved, such as the human brain with 10^{14} neurons and neuronal connections) but also their behavioral complexity (e.g., capability to adapt, perceive, move, learn, and memorize). There are two points here. One is that the kind of reductionism I favor is to a minimum set of level-independent principles, not to some elementary material unit. The other related, but more radical claim, is that we can gain new physics from the study of organisms and their behavior.

It is now well established that spatial, temporal, and functional patterns can emerge spontaneously (in a so-called self-organized fashion) in nonequilibrium physical and chemical systems (e.g., Haken, 1983). Such pattern formation is explicitly a collective phenomenon that occurs as a consequence of the interaction of a very large number of subsystems. Familiar examples include the formation of convection patterns in fluid dynamics, the emergence of the coherent light field in the laser, and the formation of concentration patterns in certain chemical reactions. Often, such patterns appear suddenly when environmental conditions are changed. The latter may be completely unspecific to the pattern that emerges (for example, when hexagons appear in Benard convection, the temperature gradient contains no information about the resulting spatial structure or its form or size). In short, there is no a priori prescription for the pattern before it arises. Instead, patterns emerge solely as a result of the dynamics of the system. (For the experts, solutions to a high-dimensional equation of motion are no longer homogeneous when a control parameter, temperature in the preceding example, crosses a critical point. Spatially patterned solutions then appear corresponding to the formation of ordered behavior.) Comparative analyses of very different experimental systems have led to the insight (which can be stated in rigorous mathematical form) that the emergence of patterns is governed by general laws that are quite independent of the material structure that realizes them.

Is it possible to understand the functional behavior of complex, biological systems in such terms? A general, across-the-board application of nonequilibrium physics to the coordinated motions of animals is hazardous (Kelso & Schöner, 1987). In contrast to certain physical systems (e.g., the laser), in biology the path from the microscopic world (e.g., the brain with all its neurons) to the essential, collective variables corresponding to macroscopic behavioral patterns is not readily accessible. In fact, in biology the definition of an appropriate microscopic level is often vague, and the collective, macroscopic state (to be derived from a microscopic description) often unknown. Nevertheless, an operational strategy may hold the key to understanding. Following is a sketch of its key features (Kelso & Schöner, 1987; Kelso, Schöner, Scholz, & Haken, 1987).

First, recognize that *understanding* depends on the language used. Inherent in the approach I advocate here (which owes much to a collaboration with the theoretical physicists Hermann Haken and Gregor Schöner and the writings of the theoretical biologist Robert Rosen) is an abstraction away from the material underpinnings of behavioral patterns. Thus, if the organizational features of living things are the primary interest, then material properties are only relevant to the extent that they support forms of organization. The aim, then, is to first identify the collective variables (or order parameters) that characterize behavioral patterns. This step is possible independent of the level of observation; the patterns of interest may be neuronal, electromyographic, kinematic, and so on. They may be characteristic of numerous functions, such as posture, reaching, walking, or talking.

Next, study the dynamics of the pattern, that is, the dynamics of the collective variables. The key step is to map observed patterns onto attractors of the collective variables (Haken, Kelso, & Bunz, 1985; Kelso & Scholz, 1985; Schöner, Haken, & Kelso, 1986), thereby allowing potentially complex behavior to be encoded into a simpler, dynamical model, whose self-consistency (postulates, assumptions) can be checked experimentally. A crucial link between theory and experiment lies in the concept of stability. Only stable, dynamic patterns can be observed; instability leads to change in pattern. There are several ways to experimentally measure stability and loss of stability (see Kelso & Scholz, 1985; Kelso et al., 1987; Scholz, Kelso, & Schöner, 1987).

Next, find control parameters that move the system through its collective states, from one pattern to another. No association with control theory, however, is implied here. Control parameters are not prescriptions for behavior; they contain no information about the details of the eventual pattern that's observed.

Once collective variables for patterned behavior are known, study the individual components and their dynamics. These lie at a lower level of description. Both the collective and component-level dynamics must be known before the former can be rigorously derived or synthesized from the latter.

In summary, understanding within the operational approach is achieved in three parts. The first involves formulating dynamical laws for observables only and making predictions that can be tested experimentally. Second is adopting a minimalist strategy, in which all consequences of a theoretical formulation are checked for their empirical validity. Only observed dynamical features should appear in any modeling; we are not interested in models that exhibit features that cannot be experimentally observed. The third part involves seeking to account for a larger number of experimental features with a smaller number of theoretical concepts.

Using the foregoing strategy (and I realize you will have to consult the sources to appreciate the full extent of its application), experimenters have shown that both stability and change of observed movement patterns emerge, in a self-organized fashion, from a relatively simple (though stochastic and nonlinear) dynamic law, that in turn can be derived from a more microscopic description (for reviews see Kelso & Schöner, 1987; Kelso et al., 1987). Moreover, recent empirical and theoretical work has led to an extension of the strategy to include perception-action patterns (Schöner & Kelso, 1988a, 1988b; Tuller & Kelso, 1985; Yamanishi, Kawato, & Suzuki, 1980) and the development of movement patterns such as walking (Thelen, Kelso, & Fogel, 1987), speech production (Kelso, Saltzman, & Tuller, 1986), and neuronal patterns (Kelso et al., 1987; Schöner & Kelso, 1988c). In addition, other directions of research are now open (for a few suggestions, see Kelso & Schöner, 1987). The citing of these references is not meant to be an advertising campaign but rather to convey the extent of the possibilities.

How did this "state of grace" evolve? The editors have asked me to provide a short autobiographical sketch, so I must comply.

Some Autobiographical Notes

In retrospect, which is notoriously fallible, my interest in the coordination of living things might seem to have been foreordained. My father was a professional footballer (U.S. readers, read soccer player) in his youth and was being touted for a Scottish international cap before a crippling knee injury led to early retirement. He never told me about his exploits on the field, in part because of modesty but more so because both my parents were dead set against my pursuing sports seriously. Grammar school was much more important. Although soccer was banned there (precisely because of its professionalism), rugby football was not. Consequently, I transferred all my early soccer skills, such as kicking with both feet, to the oblong ball. This early (and avid) interest in sports and a desire to perform them at the highest level was accompanied by two other (nearly antagonistic) main interests, namely music and drama. I entered many festivals around the country (call *Feis* in Ireland), which led to solo appearances on radio and television. Were these activities early predispositions to a future career in movement science? I doubt if they are more than coincidences.

Nevertheless, it was rugby football that took me to Canada in 1969, and 18 months later (through the encouragement of Dr. Peter Reichenbach, a professor at the University of Calgary and its rugby coach) I emigrated to Calgary, Alberta, with the intent of pursuing my studies much more seriously. To some degree I regretted not pursuing a career in medicine (which was my parents' wish), and I thought that a second chance might avail itself in Canada (which in fact it did, though again I didn't take it). Physiology and psychology were my chief interests while I was an undergraduate at Calgary, and I was fortunate with my teachers. Dr. Jerry Ells was a former student of Michael Posner at Oregon and introduced me to the new (and then quite fascinating) information-processing approach to cognitive psychology. The first real undergraduate experiment I did measured heart rate on the visual cliff in preambulatory infants. A year or so later, a similar study was published by someone else, and the results pointed to perception of depth being available earlier than the scientific community previously thought.

A course on psychomotor behavior attracted my interest in part because of a friendship that I had developed with its instructor, Dr. Barry Kerr. Kerr was a graduate of the University of Wisconsin, Madison, and encouraged me to apply there for graduate training, which I did. At Calgary I had taken full-year courses in physiology (which involved laboratory work that I enjoyed), and I developed an interest in respiratory physiology. Again, Wisconsin was the place to go, and Dr. Jerry Dempsey accepted me to work in his laboratory. However, the joint demands of course work and working in two laboratories forced me to make an early choice between physiology and motor behavior research. I chose the latter (or it chose me because that was the source of my graduate research assistantship!). Dr. George Stelmach was a relatively new professor at Wisconsin then and director of the motor behavior laboratory. He was actively engaged in research on short-term motor memory (STMM). In that first year in particular, I learned a great deal from Stelmach about the scientific (largely experimental) method. Analyses of variance, for example, had to be done by hand and the results checked by computer, so that I fully understood the mechanics of the method. I monitored the minute details of designing, setting up, and running an experiment one-on-one with George. Even so, I made errors. Lacking experience, I failed to counterbalance experimental conditions in the first study I ran for George, with the result that some 20 subjects were tested before the error was realized. There was no option but to start all over again. I never made the same mistake again. Eventually, however, the study was completed and we wrote it up for publication. Seeing my name appear as second author on the paper (Stelmach & Kelso, 1973) was a great stimulus to persevere. This experience taught me the importance of having some short-term goals, which I have emphasized with my own students.

I went through a number of identifiable (though overlapping) stages on the path to becoming a researcher (recognizing of course, that research is a process of continuous becoming, which, I hope, never really ends). The first stage is what most graduate students undergo (and it may last forever!). The strategy is to study the literature of interest, look for gaps, probe them, and then try to fill in. I do not think there is anything wrong with this bread-and-butter approach, even though it's not very creative. The nerve block work that I did with Stelmach, Wanamaker, and Wallace had that quality (Kelso et al., 1974, 1976; Kelso, Wallace, Stelmach, & Weitz, 1975). My research on visual-proprioceptive conflict with Dr. Bill Epstein arose out of his course on experimental perception, in which there was some pressure to come up with an experimentally testable idea (Kelso, Cook, Olson, & Epstein, 1975).

Stage 2, which I call asking the right kind of question, involves a little more creativity (and less fear of asking stupid questions!). For example, early in the days of STMM, I asked Stelmach why all the experiments were done with constrained movements. Because most natural movements are not like that, what if we allowed the subject to choose his or her own movements? The answer at the time was that the constrained paradigm was important to control various experimental factors (e.g., required amplitudes and starting positions). Nevertheless, an article by B. Jones (1974) retriggered my interest in the mechanisms of self-selected movement, and the result was the discovery of the preselection effect (e.g., Stelmach, Kelso, & Wallace, 1975). I remember presenting the results of our initial experiments to a visitor at the laboratory at Wisconsin and hearing his reaction—"Why didn't I think of that? It seems so obvious!" Someone quite famous, I think, defined the essence of discovery as looking at the same thing as everyone else, but seeing something different. It becomes obvious only when it is revealed!

The discovery (or rediscovery, depending on your point of view) of a temporal constraint on voluntary movements of the upper limbs followed along similar lines (Kelso, Southard, & Goodman, 1979). The initial question that arose in a graduate seminar at Iowa in early 1977 was whether Fitts's law held for two-limb movements of varying indexes of difficulty. I well remember Dan Southard—using two pieces of curtain material as targets—demonstrating that it didn't! In this case, the answer itself was less important than the way in which the answer actually emerged. The answer was only revealed when we did a high-speed film analysis of the movements—itself unusual in the motor behavior field at the time. The temporal stability that we found—in terms of the relative phasing among kinematic variables—has turned out to be a very general signature of coordination. Moreover, the insights gained through studies of interlimb coordination motivated a similar approach to understanding speech production in studies performed at Haskins Laboratories (e.g., Tuller et al., 1982; Tuller & Kelso, 1984).

Stage 3 involves my strong belief that *dynamic analogy* plays a basic role in scientific discovery and understanding. When we don't understand a phenomenon we analogize it to something we do understand (itself a step involving creative insight); this analogy, when adapted, provides a model of the phenomenon of interest. Dynamic analogy allows us to see how seemingly very different phenomena might be governed by the same kind of process. My experiments showing that the accuracy of producing terminal location was not affected much by removing feedback from the limb (Kelso, 1975) were seen as representing a style of control analogous to setting the lengths and tensions of a pair of rubber bands. Steven Keele, from the University of Oregon, first discussed this idea with me in the mid-1970s and elaborated upon it in lectures given at the University of Iowa in 1978 (see Kelso, 1982a). He saw this as a natural way to link abstractly defined targets with a mechanism for implementing them. Of course, the rubber band analogy is equivalent to the mass-spring model of Feldman (e.g., 1986) whose work was drawn to my attention by Michael Turvey. In those days, there was not much direct interaction between people doing motor behavior research and neurophysiology. It turned out, however, that experiments very similar to those I was performing on human hand movements (Kelso, 1975) were being carried out by Emilio Bizzi and colleagues on monkey head movements (Bizzi, Polit, & Morasso, 1976). Though I have not checked on the number, many further experiments have been done elucidating this style of control, which started out basically as an analogy. My view now (for what it's worth) is that all this research (taken collectively) points strongly to a functionally specific, neuromuscular organization that can be understood in terms of low-dimensional point attractor dynamics (e.g., Kelso & Tuller, 1984). That is, the patterns of behavior actually observed in targeting tasks can be mapped onto a theoretical model in which the state variables (position x, and velocity x) follow a simple dynamical law.

Dynamic analogy can only work if the behavior of the system one is trying to understand can be linked with something else whose behavior is understood. The linkage is not by virtue of shared material properties but by the fact that both share an abstract functional organization. The key insight is to recognize the functional similarity (e.g., in terms of motor equivalence or stability under perturbation) between the behavior of a living system in a given context and a corresponding dynamical system. Experimental observations are crucial, in the first place to justify the theoretical model, and in the second to check its assumptions.

I view dynamic analogy as an extremely sophisticated form of creative insight in science. Ideas, of course, do not always emerge like this. Often ideas are far more vague, at least initially. Only when one finds a specific case in which the vague notion can be given a concrete and precise meaning is it really possible to know whether the analogy is useful or not. For example, in the late 1970s, when I was working with Michael Turvey and his student (at the time) Peter Kugler, we proposed the rather general idea that a coordinative structure (a functionally specific ensemble of muscles and joints assembled as a unit) is like a dissipative structure, namely "it expresses a (marginally) stable steady state maintained by a flux of energy, that is, by metabolic processes that degrade more free energy than the drift toward equilibrium" (Kugler et al., 1980, p. 17). A Nobel prize had just been awarded in 1977 to Ilya Prigogine for his theory of dissipative structures. As a system is driven far from equilibrium it may become unstable and then evolve new (self-organized) structures showing coherent behavior. These new structures were called dissipative structures by Prigogine, and synergetic patterns by Hermann Haken (1983). When our papers were first published (Kelso et al., 1980; Kugler et al., 1980), neither the concepts of coordinative structure nor dissipative structure (see Landauer, 1981) were firmly established. In fact, it was not until the experimental discovery of a nonequilibrium phase transition in human movement that patterns of movement coordination could be understood in the language of self-organization. From this specific case, it was not only possible to make an extremely vague idea mathematically exact, but we had found a strategy through which behavioral patterns in general may be better understood (see Kelso & Schöner, 1987). Gone were the emotional connotations associated with vague and unsupported ideas. Replacing them was a rational and unifying theme that could be exactly defined. Generalization became possible by virtue of mathematical construction instead of philosophical speculation. Such is the genesis of the operational approach, in which experimentation in motor behavior and experimentation in physical theory have become intimately linked. In the future, I envisage, the coordinated motions of animals and people will become more and more a test field for a physics of the organization of living things. As Pattee (1976) says, "I do not see any way to avoid the problem of coordination and still understand the physical basis of life" (p. 171). In this regard, perhaps the most significant event in my career was the invitation by Professor Hermann Haken, Director of the Institute of Theoretical Physics, University of Stuttgart, for me to go to Stuttgart in the summer of 1984 to develop a theoretical model of phase transitions in human hand movement (Haken et al., 1985). From that point, a strategy evolved—in large part because of a close collaboration that developed with Haken—in which I saw movement coordination as a window into the dynamics of pattern formation in complex, biological systems.

There is, finally, a further state (rather than stage!) that I am somewhat hesitant to discuss. Call it imagination if you like—although I am not sure if it is not some paradoxical mixture of intuition and serendipity. Of one aspect I am sure: This state does not happen frequently. One winter's evening in 1980, late at night as I sat at my desk at Haskins Laboratories, I wondered how it might be possible to create an experimental way through which the spontaneous formation of ordered patterns might be studied. Although no one had ever studied them as such, changes in gait (e.g., trotting to galloping) were an obvious possibility. There was no way, however, I could do gait experiments in a speech laboratory where space (not to speak of subject matter) was limited. An image from a Yellow Pages advertisement cropped up, seemingly from nowhere: "Let your fingers do the walking." To my amazement, I was able to create a quadruped using the index and middle fingers of each hand! By alternating the fingers of each hand and synchronizing the middle and index fingers between the hands, I created a gait that changed spontaneously to another gait when the motions were speeded up. The effect was unbelievably compelling. Moreover, I quickly found that I could simplify the situation even more to involve the two index fingers only. Here was a paradigm that might provide a window into order-order transitions in a biological system, and I quickly established the phenomenon by running experiments on students and colleagues working at the lab.

I was fortunate that at around the same time, Professor W.J. Cunningham of Yale, who had written one of the early U.S. books on nonlinear differential equations, was teaching a course on the subject and kindly allowed Elliot Saltzman (who had come to work with me as a postdoctoral fellow) and me to participate. This experience aided me considerably in later interactions with physicists.

I formally reported the results of my phase transition experiments first in the *Bulletin of the Psychonomic Society* (Kelso, 1981) and shortly thereafter at a Kroc Foundation conference in 1982 entitled "Nonlinearities in Brain Function," organized by Arnold Mandell and Gene Yates (Kelso, 1984).

Sometime later I learned from a colleague, Dr. Diane Shapiro, that Cohen had performed a similar experiment published in a short paper in *Perceptual and Motor Skills* (L. Cohen, 1971). Thus, by the exacting standards of history, few thoughts are really new! However, Cohen's paper revealed that he had observed only transient shifts between two patterns of coordination at the wrist joints. By choosing only a single cycling frequency, he had not moved the system from one stable, collective state to another. In the language of synergetics, Cohen neither manipulated the control parameter nor characterized the coordinative patterns in terms of collective variables (order parameters) and their stability. To my knowledge—and the issue seemed important enough to deserve careful probing—Cohen never examined the issue further. Thus, the identification of a nonequilibrium phase transition in a complex, biological system had to wait another 15 years. Recently Haken (1987), in an important paper on information compression in complex systems, expressed the view that these experiments constitute "a first step [in the] important future task [of the] proper identification of order parameters and control parameters in biological systems" (p. 16). Yet the experiments would never have happened (or friends been made, a collaboration begun, and a theory developed) had I not imagined my fingers walking.

An Afterthought on Creative Juices*

The foregoing notes reveal a truism: The growth of a scientist, like the growth of a flower, must be supported by appropriate conditions throughout the growth period. I have been fortunate throughout my career that such conditions were created (despite limited resources) in the laboratories in which I worked. Specifically, I have been able to do research with only occasional (nay, to tell the truth, frequent!) constraints and requirements (e.g., write up ideas for experiments and their sequences in advance, or prepare grant proposals—a taste of real life for practicing researchers!). More important, I have had sufficient intellectual stimuli— generated from discussion, visitors, conferences, and independent study—to boost my desire to contribute something useful, if not creative. Such conditions were accompanied by a fair amount of individual drive and curiosity, not unusual among immigrants, I suppose. These seem to be the minimum conditions for a creative process to occur, be it experimentally or theoretically oriented. One of the beauties and attractions of scientific endeavor, however, is that there is no telling in advance what form the product will take.

If it is true (and we all can attest to it) that the charm of novelty is followed by the boredom of routine, then it is equally true that the creative juices must be renewed if the cycle is to continue. Thus, it is important to break existing forms of thinking—to open the mind, as it were. This becomes increasingly difficult the older and more entrenched one becomes (as I have begun to realize). Nature (and people too) seems to operate with a small set of themes. In this regard, I feel fortunate that my

---

*A colleague, J.Z. Hubert, who has worked extensively on the problem of defining creativity in science, has provoked this personal afterthought (e.g., Hubert, 1978). I outline the key aspects.

experimental work attracted the attention of scientists in different disciplines, and, as a consequence, new vistas were opened up. This affords me the possibility to create new paradigms and perhaps draw the attention of still others, including students.

It seems to me that when new ideas crop up, they attract either youth or older, more secure individuals. The establishment that runs science is, by definition almost, less open to accepting new ideas or following new paradigms. The irony is that one becomes a member of the establishment eventually, by virtue of the very activities in which one engages (editing journals, writing grants, reviewing work of peers, and publishing research). But the establishment changes too, in part because of the continuous flow of individuals through them (new degrees of freedom!). The history of science tells us that what was strange and perhaps radical in one epoch becomes established later on—after sufficient scrutiny, of course. A given view cannot sustain itself indefinitely, however. In an open system, eventually an entirely new creation emerges.

My main point is that creativity itself is a pattern that is created under appropriate conditions. The latter must be recognized and appreciated, be one a student or a professor. Whether creative thought (again, as applied to theory and/or experiment) occurs depends on (and can be predicted by) these conditions. Like coordinated action, however, its final form is not prescribed a priori or coded anywhere inside the system. Therein lies the attraction of science, in general, and the topic of coordination in particular.

ACKNOWLEDGMENTS

Some of the work discussed here was supported by a NIMH (Fundamental Neurosciences Branch) Grant MH42900-01 and a joint contract N00014-87-G-0156 from the U.S. Office of Naval Research (Physics Division and Integrated Biology Program) and the Air Force Office of Scientific Research (Artificial Neural Networks Program). I thank Dr. Betty Tuller for her comments and support over the last 14 years.

Chapter 4

Robert N. Singer

Department of Exercise and Sport Sciences
College of Health and Human Performance
University of Florida
Gainesville, Florida, U.S.A.

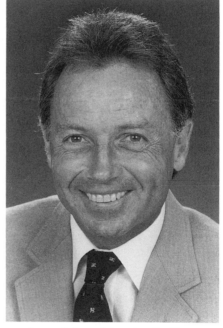

Bob Singer was born in New York City and also completed his first degree in that city, a bachelor of science in physical education from Brooklyn College in 1961. He followed this with a master's degree from Pennsylvania State University (under the supervision of John Lawther) in 1962 and a doctorate from Ohio State University in 1964 with a major in physical education and a minor in the psychology of learning. Following the completion of his graduate studies, Bob Singer held appointments in physical education at Illinois State University (1965-69), Michigan State University (1969-70), and Florida State University (1970-87). In 1987, he moved from a professorial position in the Department of Movement Science and Physical Education at Florida State University to take up his current position as chair of the Department of Exercise and Sport Sciences at the University of Florida at Gainesville.

Although Dr. Singer has published prolifically in both the motor learning and control and the sport psychology fields, his first book, *Motor Learning and Human Performance*, originally published in 1968 and now in its third edition, remains probably his most influential and best known work. This text, which was selected as one of the 20 outstanding education books of 1968 and which has now also been translated into Japanese, Korean, and German, provided the early benchmark for students of motor learning and control. Singer has since written three other books on motor learning and control, five on sport psychology, and four on physical education, many of which have been translated into foreign languages. In addition to his textbook writings, Bob Singer has maintained a very active research program.

His research work has focused upon learning from a cognitive perspective, and original contributions to knowledge have arisen from his experimental work on information-processing capabilities, learner strategies, and attentional processes (e.g., Singer, 1978a, 1980; Singer & Gerson, 1981; Singer, Hagenbeck, & Gerson, 1981). Singer's research interests appear more diverse than those of Henry and Kelso and are driven more by the need to generate knowledge on practical, applied issues than by the need to exhaustively test generic theories of movement control. His research interests extend to questions relating to motivation and performer readiness (e.g., Rudisill & Singer, 1988; Singer & McCaughan, 1978), and his experimental contributions in this field make him (like Carron, chapter 10) an important link between the fields of motor learning and control and sport psychology. Bob Singer has a very high-profile professional involvement in sport psychology, particularly at the international level, and he was honored by the International Society of Sport Psychology in 1989 in recognition of his contribution to the work of that body. He was elected president of their Society for 4-year terms in 1985 and 1989. Earlier, Dr. Singer was invited to serve on the first Sports Medicine Council of the U.S. Olympic Committee as the coordinator of the sport psychology area. Recently, he was selected by his peers as one of the top 10 sport psychologists of the past decade (Straub, 1991). In 1989, he was also ranked among the 10 most notable contemporary physical educators in the United States (Edwards, 1989), due largely to his joint contributions in the motor learning and control and sport and exercise psychology fields. That same year, Singer was given the Distinguished Alumnus Award by Brooklyn College. Professor Singer has been an editorial board member of a number of journals in the human action field including *Journal of Motor Behavior, Research Quarterly for Exercise and Sport, Journal of Sport and Exercise Psychology, International Journal of Sport Psychology, The Sport Psychologist,* and *Journal of Applied Sport Psychology.*

In this chapter, Bob Singer guides us through the development of his research career and his transition from an unfocused to a focused program of experimentation on cognitive processes and learner strategies. In reading his contribution, consider the information-processing framework in which his work has developed, and compare and contrast this with the orientation of Henry and especially with the one proposed by Kelso. Note Singer's continued use of paradigms taken directly from experimental psychology and his application of these imported ideas to the unique problems posed by the learning of movement skills. Also, note carefully his eclectic interests and use of parallel research programs. Above all, as with Henry and Kelso, learn from his commitment to, and enthusiasm for, the use of experimentation to uncover important elements within the motor learning and control field.

AUTOBIOGRAPHY

It is difficult to know where to start. Or what to remember. Or even how to remember with accuracy those thoughts that led to events, which in turn led to outcomes, which in turn led to other thoughts, which . . .

The Early Years

Perhaps it might be helpful to offer a brief perspective of my doctoral experiences, as a starting point. In 1962 I decided on an area of specialization, but after 6 months I realized there was a lack of harmony between this specialization and me. What to do? I wasn't excited about existing options. It just so happened that on occasion I would play tennis with D.D. Wickens, a famous classical conditioning psychologist. We discussed my interest in the psychology of learning as applied to motor skills.

Only about five universities on the continent offered courses in motor learning at that time. This area (as well as sport psychology) had not yet been defined in departments of physical education, or any other department for that matter. Certain individuals stood out, however, who were conducting research on motor learning topics: Henry at the University of California, Berkeley; Slater-Hammel at the University of Indiana; and Lawther at Pennsylvania State University, who was my adviser at the master's level in 1961-62.

I was allowed to create my own doctoral curriculum at the Ohio State University. In every course I took in psychology, most notably Leslie Brigg's course, entitled Human Performance (a course with a promising title but with surprisingly different and more complicated material than I expected), I kept two sets of notes. One was directly related to the course content; the other included my thoughts as to how any research or theory could apply to physical education and sport settings or to understanding of the learning of skills and how to teach more effectively. Every topic seemed to excite me, from problems dealing with the transfer of skills to practice trade-off conditions (e.g., speed vs. accuracy) to the emerging area of cognitive psychology. Information-processing, cybernetic, hierarchical control models, spawned in the 1940s, were a welcome relief to traditional behavioristic approaches with which researchers attempted to explore the learner/performer's functional capabilities and to understand the demands of various types of tasks. I couldn't wait to start researching various topics.

Because I never really had a doctoral adviser (I was basically on my own), my program was unstructured and I completed a variety of courses. No one ever guided me in the research process or taught me how to think systematically in exploring one particular issue or related issues. My earlier research publications reflected this state of affairs. After graduation in 1964, I published 14 articles in *The Research Quarterly** from 1965 to 1969, on a wide range of topics. Typically, I used athletic skills such as fencing (speed-accuracy trade-off effects) and archery (transfer effects related to initial task degree of difficulty) in the motor learning studies. I undertook a few studies with children on the going-togetherness of physical, perceptual-motor, and academic achievement variables. Personality differences between and within baseball and tennis players were the topic of another investigation.

There was no unified comprehensive body of scholarly literature in motor learning or sport psychology at that time. Cratty attempted to create such a body in 1964, and I tried to go a step further by writing a motor learning text in 1968, *Motor Learning and Human Performance*, which was recognized as one of the top 20 books published in education that year. Nevertheless, my own research publications reflected the lack of a cohesive body of knowledge and a sufficient base of literature as well as my own proclivity to become excited in one problem area after another. Ideas would come to me as I read studies in psychological journals, and I would attempt to design a study with gross motor activities that could increase understanding of certain phenomena or could benefit instructional approaches. It was quite a shotgun approach, in retrospect, an approach that I soon changed.

Sport psychology was officially introduced to North America in 1968 with the formation of the North American Society for the Psychology of Sport and Physical Activity. Studies on topics related to sport psychology were in evidence for many years prior to that date, however. It was difficult to differentiate between motor learning and sport psychology in those days (and perhaps still is today). I tried to overview the field of sport psychology in 1972, with the publication of *Coaching, Athletics, and Psychology*. The way I approached motor learning, from an applied motor-learning perspective, was very much related to concerns in sport psychology as to how individuals involved in sport could learn and perform

---

*Complete sources as well as reference to many of my publications are omitted. Many of the more important publications are presented in the reference list of this book.

effectively. But it wasn't until 1975, 11 years and many publications following my PhD, that I fully charted a unified course of action for my research as well as my doctoral students.

The Focused Years

My approach evolved as I began analyzing cognitive processes involved in motor learning and performance. At that time, my serious scholarly colleagues in motor learning were drawn to the motor control area. Research on academic questions concerning motor programming and related topics were being addressed in the laboratory with simple motor tasks. But I was interested in understanding information processing and related mental processes associated with the learning and performing of real-world complex motor acts, such as in sport. I felt that such activities were much more complicated and engaged the learner/performer's cognitive processes in a highly involved manner. But how? What should be studied and in what way? As an aside, and as I reflect back to the early and mid-1970s, I have always been fascinated with factors that contribute to achievement in motor skills, especially the roles of various cognitive processes. Personal interests led me to establish a number of guidelines in my work, which I can verbalize more effectively today than I could years ago. Perhaps these guidelines explain my scholarly directions during the years:

- To determine the nature and role of cognitive processes in the learning of motor skills as well as achievement reflected by high levels of performance
- To identify strategies that can be used to improve the functioning of these processes and in turn influence achievement
- To analyze the self-motivation to persist and achieve, while being personally satisfied in the process, and to determine personal strategies to accomplish this process
- To generalize findings to all motor skills, in a generic sense, but with a special thrust toward athletic skills
- To contribute to scholarly and professional developments in motor learning, pedagogy in general, and sport psychology, realizing commonalties in my work among these areas as well as unique considerations
- To design laboratory research that could advance a body of knowledge as well as improve instruction and facilitate learning and performance
- To undertake interesting and novel research and create contemporary topical areas rather than become routinized, repetitive, and engaged in traditional research topics

One of the first approaches with which I used these ideas was in determining what happened when learners could freely use their cognitive processes in learning a primary task and a related one. I compared this discovery group to a group that was highly prompted and guided in the first task. Neither group received instructions for the second task. I engineered the idea for a procedural laboratory task called the serial manipulation apparatus. It was computer managed, had a visual display, and used many varied response manipulanda. The subjects had to learn an appropriate sequence of responses to a particular signal and were evaluated for a criterion of accuracy. Many real-world activities involve a series of steps that must be performed in the right sequences if the total act is to be considered acceptable. People must learn how to attend to cues and organize their responses systematically and quickly.

The focus in this study was not achievement in the first task. We (my student Lee Gaines and I) expected the prompted group to outperform the discovery group. We were particularly interested in transfer to the second task. Which group would gain more from learning the first task and would then fare better in the second task? We hypothesized the discovery group, and we were right. Apparently, learners who are actively involved in the learning process pick up more information and, although slower in learning at first, ultimately achieve more in related task situations. The article was published in the *American Educational Research Journal*. Subsequently, Dale Pease (one of my students) and I explored other questions concerning transfer and retention with similar groups of subjects and published the results in 1976 and 1978 in the *Research Quarterly for Exercise and Sport*.

In these studies we determined the results that occurred when we left learners alone. Apparently, they could develop strategies that facilitated the acquisition of a transfer task. But then I thought, what would happen if instead of leaving learners alone we attempted to teach them task-relevant strategies? Shouldn't there be ways to help learners learn how to learn? If we could understand more about various cognitive processes that seem to work in sequence or in parallel, perhaps then we might be able to determine which strategies should enhance the functioning of these processes. We needed to design experiments to test our hypotheses.

Cognitive Processes and Learner Strategies

Of great interest to me during the 1970s was the advancement of cognitive psychology and the attempt to refine knowledge about the information-processing capabilities of people and the types of strategies (especially those related to memory) that could be particularly useful in facilitating learning and performance in achievement-oriented tasks. To what degree could strategies studied in the learning of classroom matter be applied to movement-oriented activities, especially those requiring the production of skill? Which types of strategies are unique to those movement activities? And how should these activities be categorized conveniently, in order to delineate more precise strategies related to achievement? This whole area excited me, because I felt that it was virtually untapped and yet was quite important from a variety of perspectives.

A milestone in my thinking occurred in 1977 when I was invited to be the only scholar representing the skills area to participate in a major conference entitled "Learning Strategies: Measures and Modules," sponsored by the Defense Advanced Research Projects Agency (DARPA). My invited paper, "Cognitions, Strategies, and Motor Behavior," required me to search through a wide assortment of articles, to organize my thinking, and to speculate about what was known and what should be known. From the experiences of developing and presenting this paper (which later became a chapter in a book edited by O'Neil, who organized the conference), hearing papers representing other disciplines, and exchanging ideas with respected scholars, I generated a major proposal that was funded by DARPA from 1977 to 1980. The grant provided me with ample resources and time to think.

For the first phase, I tried to conceptualize a model of motor behavior that emphasized the potential sequences and parallel operations of various cognitive processes. I later identified alternative strategies that might enhance the functioning of these processes. I speculated a great deal about the basis of theories and research primarily associated with the learning of cognitive matter, because very little was available in the motor behavior literature. Then, I developed a series of laboratory tasks (some computer managed) to compare the effectiveness of different types of learning strategies. One task was the serial manipulation apparatus (SMA), described briefly in this chapter and in detail in a 1975 *Journal of Motor Behavior* article. Besides undertaking this procedural task, I created a visual tracking task in which subjects had to learn to track a wave form (with variations in structure and speed in presentation) as displayed on an oscilloscope. A linear positioning task was also used, with various location points to be recalled.

In a few studies with the positioning task, for example, my students and I compared such strategies as imagery, labeling, irrelevant labeling, and kinesthetic awareness; we also used a control (no strategy). Imagery was the most productive strategy. We identified other strategies and compared them with other tasks. From a perspective completely different from the learning strategy one, in other research we examined strategies associated with motivation, expectations, and attributions, and we looked at the influences of these strategies on learning. We felt that motivational strategies associated with self-perceptions could strongly affect achievement.

During this phase of experimentation, we intuitively formulated strategies. It became apparent that we needed a stronger approach in our research. A major review and conceptual article that I published in the *Research Quarterly for Exercise and Sport* in 1981 with one of my students, Richard Gerson, helped to suggest some future directions. We developed a task classification scheme within an information-processing perspective considering input properties, response demands, and feedback availability. This scheme provided guidelines for the determination of strategies for a particular task categorization. At the same time, I reconsidered material I had written in the late 1970s concerning the general applicability of strategies, from one task or context to another. The question I raised was, Does each strategy have to be taught specific to a particular task? Are there strategies, and ways of teaching them, that might transfer, or generalize, to a number of learning/performance situations? Influencing the learning process this way, if possible, would certainly save instructional program time and would help the learners at times when instructors are not present.

The Generalizability of Strategies

At that point in my thinking, I was aware of developments in cognitive psychology in memory and the concept of metamemory (learning how to remember and how to monitor memory effectiveness) as introduced by Flavell, and I knew of self-regulatory processes that could be useful in a variety of stress-provoking situations (e.g., Meichenbaum, 1977). However, I did not tie the concepts of metacognitions and metastrategies (higher order strategies useful to learners across a number of situations, such as how to concentrate, monitor progress, and learn efficiently) to my own work until a few years after I designed an ambitious program that I labeled "strategy generality."

Simply put, the hypothesis was that such strategies (which I later termed metastrategies) could be identified and techniques could be advanced as to how best to teach them. The best instructional program, I reasoned, teaches learners strategies for analyzing tasks, situations, and themselves so learners can apply those strategies on their own in subsequent achievement-oriented situations. A successful program should stimulate people to self-initiate appropriate strategies.

A major design we have used in our research is formulation of an initial (primary) learning task, with which experimental subjects are provided with relevant learning strategies, whereas a control group is not. All subjects attempt to learn not only the primary task but one or more related tasks as well. The effectiveness of strategy instruction in the primary task as well as its transferability to another task has been demonstrated in a few investigations. As we obtain answers to the more general questions, many other questions are raised in the process. Should strategies be taught in the context of one task or in a context-free or multicontext situation?

What are the boundaries (types of information-processing demands) of tasks within which a particular strategy can be expected to be useful? To borrow the concept of motor schema, which is typically associated with the nature of motor program control, are there strategy schemata?

The discussion thus far has been on strategies that may be effective for all learners. But distinct personal cognitive styles (ways of approaching learning) have been identified in the literature. We have begun to examine some dimensions, such as the impulsivity-reflectivity one. If a learner tends to be ineffectively reactive or overly pensive, can he or she be provided with strategies to overcome such a performance limitation? Results in our 1985 study were quite favorable in this regard. Other relevant styles need to be determined along with prominent strategies for a style that is undesirable for a particular type of task.

Speaking of task considerations, our strategy research has been primarily directed toward brief self-placed (closed) skills. These occur in a stable environment with a fixed situation. The person has time to preview, prepare, and act when ready. Examples in sport are serving a volleyball or tennis ball, stroking a golf ball, and executing a dive. Such acts, although quite complex and difficult to accomplish with great proficiency, nevertheless lend themselves more easily to analysis than do externally paced skills. (This is the primary reason for studying them almost exclusively until now.) Externally paced activities usually involve uncertainty, anticipation, and rapid decision making, because the person is paced by an opponent's and/or an object's action. We have begun to study strategies associated with improving such processes. A grant received from the United States Tennis Association is allowing us to analyze information processing processes (i.e., visual search, anticipation, decision-making, and response preparation related to player quickness). The trainability of these processes will also be determined.

The Five-Step Strategy

I began to realize that virtually all experimental strategy research tends to be singular (i.e., one strategy's effectiveness is determined in one study). And yet, in real life, skilled performers use a number of complementary strategies. It's as if these performers have packaged themselves to generate a series of successful internal operations, depending on the demands and length of the challenging activity.

My observations of and interactions with many top athletes in many self-paced sports, observations made by colleagues, and biographical and autobiographical reports of athletes all reveal a similar series of internal operations that occur. Successful athletes have mastered strategies to create an optimal operational medium. From this information, I designed what I have called the five-step strategy for self-paced skills. Each of the steps, or substrategies, has been investigated quite extensively and singularly by others, indicating the important roles these steps play in influencing learning and performance. Therefore, I speculated that the five-step strategy should help beginners acquire skills rapidly in any self-paced activity as well as help more advanced athletes to perform well with a high degree of regularity. The steps are

- Readying
- Imaging
- Focusing
- Executing
- Evaluating

The first substrategy, readying, assists the learner in attaining an optimal preparatory mental-physical state to perform. The second substrategy, imaging, calls for the person to create a mental picture of the subsequent movement as it should be performed, thus establishing a positive set for performance. The third substrategy, focusing, encourages selective and exclusive attention to one relevant feature of the stimulus object so that irrelevant thoughts are blocked out. The fourth substrategy, executing, guides the individual to trigger the act as if it were automatic, without conscious activity toward performance. Finally, the fifth substrategy, evaluating, requires the learner to assess the performance outcome as well as the effectiveness of each previous substrategy in contributing to the performance level.

We have designed a series of experiments to determine the effectiveness of the strategy, using novel gross motor tasks administered in a laboratory setting. We are in the process of testing the strategy on the learning of the tennis serve and the racquetball serve. The first investigation, conducted by Singer and Suwanthada (1986), demonstrated that the five-step strategy taught on one occasion in various contexts and under different conditions facilitated the acquisition rate of and performance level in three novel self-paced tasks. The strategy apparently can generalize across learning tasks. Subsequent research (Singer, DeFrancesco, & Randall, 1989; Singer, Flora, & Abourezk, 1989) has yielded confirming data.

This type of research nicely ties together scholarly literature and information with practical ramifications for teachers and students, coaches and athletes, and learners of self-paced activities in general. Indeed, the process of learning can be enhanced when learners acquire and apply relevant strategies. As is the case with many research programs, many questions arise that seem worthy of pursuit. For example, we are attempting to answer the following:

- Which are the most favorable contexts and conditions for strategy instruction that will lead to the best results for learners who will attempt to master a number of self-paced activities?

- When is the best point of introduction of a learning strategy: before any direct task experience, after a limited experience, or after substantial experience?
- Considering developmental factors, what is the youngest age at which a subject can learn a strategy and apply it appropriately to a number of tasks?

Such questions are relevant for understanding the effectiveness of the five-step strategy or any other learning strategy, whether a strategy is taught as a task-specific learning/performance strategy or as a meta-strategy to generalize across tasks. Research with the highly skilled is more difficult to undertake. However, my personal experience with the highly skilled has been quite rewarding, because proficient athletes in such sports as golf, basketball, and tennis seem to feel that the five-step strategy strengthens their performance potential in their specialized sports. It will be nice if scientific data bear out our assumptions.

Besides exploring strategies for self-paced acts, we are now exploring strategies that promote achievement in externally paced acts. The five-step strategy (rather, the first four steps) can probably be used in these activities, if the action is slow enough and there is sufficient time to preview the situation. This occurs, for example, when the person is all alone for a jump shot in basketball. There is time to get set, image, focus, and execute. The faster the action, the less time there is to ready, image, and even focus attention in a desirable manner. Key strategies in externally paced activities appear to be related to the allocation and direction of attention (depending on demands at any moment), anticipation, and rapid but effective decision making. We hope to determine to what extent individuals can be trained to use such processes for specific skills, and indeed, to what degree strategies learned can transfer to other externally paced tasks.

Additional Perspectives

I have chosen to concentrate on explaining my interests and research developments in regard to cognitive processes, learning strategies, and achievement in motor skills. But through the years, in fact, I have become engaged in a wide variety of projects. It has been challenging as well as fun to be a part of many of the developments in motor learning and sport psychology.

On many occasions I have been asked to speculate about future directions in these fields, practical instructional or intervention techniques, and other matters. The varied projects have required me to expand my knowledge base and my perspectives. The challenges, although demanding, take away the potential boredom of working in a highly specialized area over a long period of time.

Besides some isolated research thrusts, an area of particular interest to me is an individual's motivation to persist and achieve while gaining personal satisfaction in the process. My doctoral students and I have undertaken a number of experiments examining the interactive role of expectancies and attributions in persistence and performance. We have administered various strategies in order to ascertain cause-effect relationships. We have also looked at other self-perceptions, such as self-concept.

To me, the cognitive motivational area is as exciting as the learning strategies area. We all need to acquire strategies to improve our information-processing processes, as well as to motivate ourselves to continue with an activity, practice well, and realize our achievement potential. Preferably, we can learn to initiate such strategies at the proper time. The goal is effective self-management and perceptions of control over self and circumstances. Any research that furthers our understanding in this area—especially concerning our abilities to generate strategies to feel in control, to learn, to be optimally and continually motivated, and to feel fulfilled in the process—should be of great benefit to instructors, athletes, and learners of all kinds.

As I review the orientation and direction of my projects, they appear to be quite global and ambitious. However, I would like to make a few comments on my approach, acknowledging that I have never felt that I've come close to what I would like to accomplish. The following are my goals, which are reflected in my working style:

- To be sincerely interested in whatever I undertake and to appreciate the scientific process, effort, commitment, and achievement
- To be continually intellectually active, a desire that can be attributed to dedicated colleagues and to challenging and conscientious graduate students with whom I have been fortunate to interact, and with whose presence I hope I will be blessed again and again in the future
- To read and write during many evenings, nights, and weekends, and to look forward to those quiet and generally productive times
- To be aware of research published in a variety of fields that might lend me a more interdisciplinary, integrated, "big-picture" approach to my understandings, and to interact with scholars from these fields

Many students and others starting out in motor learning and sport psychology often are dismayed by the lack of a strong and extensive body of literature, standard and standardized research paradigms, sufficient practical information, and clear guidelines as to what the field of motor behavior is all about and how to progress in it. Yes, we can be disappointed and even frustrated with such limitations. A road that is not well paved and lit is not easy to follow. In fact, it could be a dead end.

The optimistic view is that it is exciting to be part of the process of constructing paths and directions. Thus, there are no limitations, only challenges. We are not as constrained as those working in more established areas. We don't have the convenience of following a well-traveled road requiring little thought, but we can experience feelings of exhilaration associated with exploration, problem solving, and taking important steps in formulating a substantive body of knowledge.

I'm reminded of the story of a pair of young twins, one an optimist and the other a pessimist. Scientists decided to study their behaviors in detail and placed them in separate cubicles. The pessimistic twin was analyzed first.

Upon examination of the pessimistic twin's chamber, the scientists saw many play objects, and yet the subject looked very dejected. One scientist asked, "With such a fine looking ten-speed bicycle, how could you be so unhappy?" The twin answered, "I'd try to ride it and probably hurt myself!" "But what about that neat baseball glove?" another scientist queried. "I'd probably lose it," the twin responded. "And how about that fancy train set?" was another question. The twin replied, "I'd probably break it trying to put it together."

The scientists went to the other chamber. The optimistic twin seemed very happy, even though no objects were located in the chamber. The only unusual substance present was a pile of horse manure! The twin was digging enthusiastically. "What are you doing, and how come you're so happy?" a scientist asked. The twin responded cheerfully, "Oh, with all this manure, there must be a horse here somewhere."

An incredible number of interesting questions in the motor behavior area need to be resolved, and any would-be researcher should be thrilled with this prospect. Furthermore, motor performance data can be recorded conveniently and frequently. This is not true with cognitive and affective behaviors. The ability to evaluate motor performance data is a strong asset in the designing of research and in the ability of the researcher to collect meaningful data that can be analyzed conveniently in statistical terms. In addition, more journals are being produced in recent years to accommodate the growing interest in generating and reading about research in motor learning and sport psychology.

I hope that you feel the way I do. If you do, stop wasting your time. Put down this book (after reading all of it, of course) and see if you can't design an interesting study—interesting to you as well as to others. Once you get started, you won't stop.

Chapter 5

H.T.A. (John) Whiting

Department of Psychology
University of York
York, England

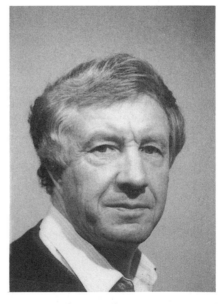

Born in London in 1929, John Whiting gained a teacher's certificate from the University of Nottingham in 1952 and a diploma of physical education from Loughborough College in 1953. After holding various teaching appointments in physical education, he obtained a lectureship in physical education at the University of Leeds in 1960 and soon thereafter commenced part-time postgraduate study in the Department of Psychology at the same institution. A keen squash player, Whiting completed a master of arts degree in psychology in 1964 and a PhD in experimental psychology in 1967 (under the supervision of Dr. Dennis Holding). His doctoral work (some of which is described in this chapter) focused on the learning of ball skills and provided the basis for his best known work, the influential 1969 text, *Acquiring Ball Skill: A Psychological Interpretation*. *Acquiring Ball Skill* gave experimentation in the motor learning and control field an applied orientation that had been

This chapter was written when the author was at the Faculty of Human Movement Sciences, The Free University, Amsterdam, The Netherlands.

absent from the field since the ergonomics-inspired work of the 1930s and 1940s.

The orientation of Whiting's work was, in fact, so different from the narrow, laboratory-based testing of simple theories of motor control that dominated both motor learning and control and experimental psychology at the time that the significance of his work took a long time to become established both in his native England (as his autobiographical chapter reveals) and in North America. Indeed, it has only been with the recent resurgence in interest in natural skills (especially catching), inspired by Gibson's (1979) ecological psychology, that much of John Whiting's pioneering work on ball skills has been accorded the recognition it deserves.

Whiting's contribution to the development of the motor learning and control field in England draws very strong parallels to Franklin Henry's contribution in North America, despite their obvious differences in applied versus basic research focus. Like Henry, Whiting, through excellence in experimentation, was able to establish the academic credibility of research conducted within physical education. In many respects, Dr. Whiting's achievement in this regard is greater than Henry's because Whiting used an applied research focus rather than an approach that to some degree mimicked the already accepted methods of mainstream psychology. Again, like Henry's work, Whiting's research activity was quick to attract graduate students (such as John Alderson, Bob Sharp, Frank Sanderson, Ian Cockerill, and Dave Tyldesley) who furthered the cause of applied research on ball skills, especially catching (e.g., Alderson & Whiting, 1974; Sanderson & Whiting, 1978; Sharp & Whiting, 1974; Tyldesley & Whiting, 1975; Whiting & Cockerill, 1972).

Indeed, the 1970s work from Whiting's group in Leeds still clearly represents, in the history of the motor learning and control field, the golden age of experimentation on ball skills. The parallels with Henry also continue in terms of John Whiting's contributions to the profession and his contribution to the understanding of research topics outside of his ball skills focus. In the 1970s he edited a number of state-of-the-art summaries of applied motor learning and control literature (Whiting, 1972, 1975a, 1975c, 1975d), published a blueprint for the formation of an academic discipline of human movement studies (Brooke & Whiting, 1973), and initiated (in 1975) a publication that became a vehicle for experimentation in the discipline—the *Journal of Human Movement Studies*. He also published occasional papers on a range of topics in the sport and exercise psychology field and in the movement impairment/rehabilitation area.

Whiting moved to the Netherlands in 1977 to become professor and head of the Department of Psychology in the Faculty of Human Movement Sciences at Free University, Amsterdam. Along with colleagues and graduate students, he continued his experimentation on ball skills and motor learning in this new environment, but his work markedly shifted in theoretical orientation away from cognitive, information-processing views to the ecological, dynamical perspective arising out of the writings of Gibson (1979) on perception and Bernstein (1967) on action.

During his period in Amsterdam, Whiting initiated, and today remains editor of, the very successful journal *Human Movement Science*. He also edited and published a very influential text that reprinted and reassessed the works of Bernstein (Whiting, 1984). Whiting also, with Mike Wade, edited two landmark texts in which the theoretical debates between the cognitive and dynamical perspectives of motor learning and control were directed to the issues posed by motor development (Wade & Whiting, 1986; Whiting & Wade, 1986). John Whiting "retired" in 1989 with the title of professor emeritus from The Free University in Amsterdam, The Netherlands, and accepted an honorary professorship in the psychology department at the University of York, in England.

John Whiting has made, and continues to make, enduring contributions to motor learning and control research on issues related to catching, motor learning, and the theory of human movement (see van Wieringen & Bootsma, 1989, for a tribute and a collection of selected papers). He has persistently shown the value of examining natural actions and the importance of addressing issues of learning in addition to the predominant focus on questions of control (e.g., Whiting, 1980, 1982). In reading this chapter, note, among other things, the role of chance factors in molding his research career; his willingness to undertake data-driven research; the resistance he encountered early in his career because his approach did not adhere to the dominant, reductionist, laboratory-based approach of the time; and the plasticity in his theoretical views, in particular, his willingness to reeducate and reorient his theoretical perspective late in his research career.

AUTOBIOGRAPHY

On the face of it, a request to put one's whole experimental career in the area of motor skill into perspective, particularly when it spans a period of almost 30 years, seems something of a tall order. Surprisingly, this did not prove to be the case, events that shaped my career being almost as clear to me now as at the time they occurred. Perhaps this is because major turning points are related to those significant others who, in the main, account for developments in one's career that are other than fortuitous. This still leaves much room for fortuity! If I had not chosen to study physical education, if in the 3rd year of my study the first student research position at Loughborough had not become available, if after I spent 6 years teaching physical education a position for a lecturer at Leeds University had not become open—the list could be extended!

Because up to the age of 20 I had never had plans to study or teach physical education, my arrival in the profession must in itself be fortuitous. This career move was precipitated during my period of military service as a consequence of my friendship with Peter Simons, who had already been accepted to study physical education at Loughborough College. He not only put the idea of entering the field into my head but also persuaded me (against my better judgment at the time) that it was a viable proposition.

The validity of my choice was confirmed during my stay at Loughborough—I was in my element. Although the practical involvement, particularly to someone who at that time could make no claim to athletic superiority, was in itself fulfilling, I had to wait until my final year of study for real fulfillment. Fortuitously, from my point of view, George Highmore had at that time (1952) joined the education staff at Loughborough, having recently (although rather belatedly due to war service) completed a PhD thesis entitled *Factorial Analysis of Athletic Ability*. He provided the opportunity and the inspiration—for the first time at Loughborough—for a small group of students to be involved in a follow-up study in the same area. I became so intrigued with the question of the factorial structure of athletic ability and the excitement of the research atmosphere that I devoted the greater part of my final year to this enterprise. As a consequence, an interest in individual differences has pervaded my career, and, although it plays no central role, I return to the theme from time to time (e.g., Jansen & Whiting, 1984). A complete commitment was, at that time, also necessary for any real accomplishment. These were days of innocence—before computers, before calculators (for Loughborough anyway!), and before refined analytical techniques. Only those who have completed a factor analysis by hand will appreciate the level of that commitment! To this day, my mind is quite likely to become momentarily occupied with topics like Aitken's method of pivotal condensation or Holzinger's bi-factor method. I had the satisfaction that the work stemming from my (minor) thesis was eventually published (following a more sophisticated reanalysis at the University of London) in the *British Journal of Statistical Psychology* (Highmore & Taylor, 1954). In no small way, this provided the incentive to go on.

Although the need to take up a position teaching physical education occupied my early years (1953-60), research and further study were never far from my mind. During my first teaching appointment—through the grace and foresight of the headmaster George Irving—I was able to continue my investigations, this time into forecasting the gymnastic ability of schoolboys. Although I never brought this work to a very satisfactory conclusion, it was sufficient to merit the award of the very modest Wortley Research Prize of the University of Nottingham in 1956. In the same year

my career orientation necessitated a move to another and different type
of school, which, in turn, necessitated a curtailing of my research interests.
It was only toward the end of my stay in that school (1959) that I became
itchy footed—missing the academic stimulation. From then onward, the
pace quickened! I registered for an external degree in statistics with the
University of London and, shortly thereafter, changed to a degree in
psychology. To this day I'm not sure precisely why I chose psychology,
although it undoubtedly had something to do with my interest in skill
learning (which developed during my research enterprise at Loughborough) and my increasing commitment, since that time, to team sport.

The Leeds Connection

Late in 1959, I was confronted by an advertisement for a lecturer in
physical education at Leeds University. Although at that time I had little
idea what such a position involved, the reference to research (albeit in
small print!) was a sufficient trigger. I obtained the position at a university
that was to be my home for the next 17 years. I confirmed later that my
(limited) research experience was the telling factor in my appointment—all
had not been in vain! Not only did this appointment require a change of
orientation in my teaching life, it also forced me to consider the viability
of completing the external degree for which I was registered. Fortuitously,
at that time Pat Meredith, chairman of the department of psychology at
Leeds, was busy with the development of a part-time master of arts degree
(by examination) for a limited number of mature students. It seemed that
I had made the appropriate decisions en route and was accepted as a
student. Completion of this part-time master's degree within a 4-year
period required considerable commitment, and research had to take a
secondary position. The little research I was able to carry out between
1960 and 1964 continued the individual differences tradition. One of my
tasks in the Department of Physical Education was the teaching of adult
nonswimmers. An extended experience with this population led me to
predict personality differences between persistent nonswimmers and
those who learned to swim comparatively quickly. This research led to a
number of publications and ultimately to my second book (Whiting, 1970),
Teaching the Persistent Non-Swimmer.

Immediately following the completion of my master's degree, I registered for a PhD in the area of experimental psychology—and thus cur-
tailed, for a period, my interest in individual differences. This choice
was not altogether fortuitous; Dennis Holding had recently joined the
psychology department at Leeds and was willing to act as my supervisor.
My topic area was fairly easy to choose. My interest in ball skills was
confirmed by both my teaching program and my own personal playing
experience. I had for a long time been intrigued with statements made by

teachers of ball skills that were seldom backed by empirical evidence. One of the most universal of these was the instruction "keep your eye on the ball"! This, together with the relative lack of attention to input characteristics in skill acquisition in the literature at that time, induced me to pursue this issue empirically. However, the methodology I should employ was unclear. I always remember Holding pointing out to me two extreme methods of approach. I could, following an extensive literature review, come up with a proposal for a critical experiment to decide upon the merits of conflicting theoretical positions, or I could simply give nature a prod and see how it reacted! I chose the latter, and I note, in retrospect, that I seem to have persisted in that vein!

What is perhaps more surprising, given the literature on skill at that time, was that I should choose a task (catching and throwing, albeit in a laboratory setting) that had at least a semblance of what Neisser (1976) later termed ecological validity. The major problem in that research was instrumentation, a problem with which I was frequently confronted in the years that followed, because my own department had no technical support. This meant in essence that all apparatuses had to be conceived and made by myself or, later, by my research students. Whether we would have progressed further with more technical support remains an open question; I am doubtful. Real life questions inevitably lead to creativity in apparatus design and methodology. (Figure 5.1 is a classic example of solving a difficult problem by relatively "Heath Robinson," but effective apparatuses. It remains my favorite.) To this day, I remain convinced that researchers can provide meaningful answers to important research questions using relatively unsophisticated apparatuses and approaches. To give a further example, the apparatus used for most of my PhD (Whiting, 1967) experiments was a development of the pub-skittles game euphemistically called "devil-among-the-tailors." A newspaper report in which this apparatus was cited invoked negative reactions from some quarters—including a telephone call from a person asking me (in a derogatory way) who had funded such research! I like to think that the contribution to the skills literature was more positively appraised.

A major problem for me at that time was the feeling that I was plowing a lone field—there were few people, outside my own research students, with whom I could discuss my work in any meaningful way. The problem was signaled in the comments of a reviewer of one of my (successful) grant applications to the Social Science Research Council, who suggested that the applicant would benefit from having closer contact with other academic psychologists working in similar areas. On that point, I was in agreement, but the further suggestion that I should switch my research interests in other directions in the future (with the hint that this might better justify funding) was not only not appreciated but was not followed.

This isolated position was, however, soon to change. Shortly after I completed my PhD (1967), my book *Acquiring Ball Skill: A Psychological*

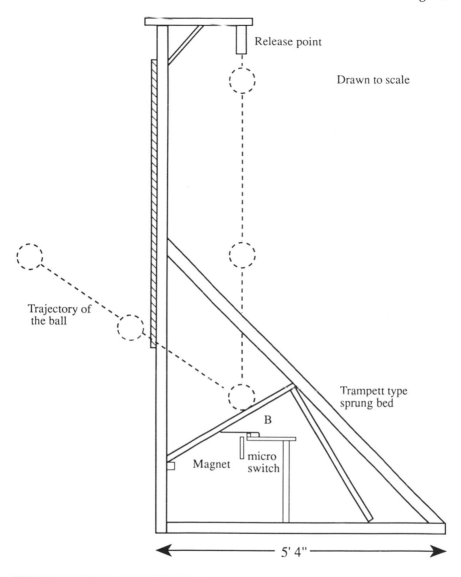

Figure 5.1 Ball-dropping gantry.

Interpretation was published (Whiting, 1969), giving me access to a wider international community of scientists and the opportunity to travel and to discuss my ideas in many countries. Although I have been trying to write a second edition for some years with a completely changed orientation, the book is still published in its original form to this day. In the meantime my ideas have changed, although it is not altogether clear if they have moved on! My position became less isolated also due to an influx of research students into my department to work on my projects. Because of my PhD work and interests, it is perhaps inevitable that these students opted for topics like input characteristics of ball skill acquisition, hand-eye coordination, dynamic visual acuity, and the development of velocity perception.

Leeds to Amsterdam—*Enkel Reis**

The 17 years I spent at Leeds were significant years, in which not only my own research career was fostered, but the department, small as it was, built up a very good national and international reputation. However, success in itself—as indexed by scientific publications and attraction of postgraduate students and visiting scholars—is not necessarily the criterion that universities adopt in planning their future academic development (although such criteria may be quickly invoked when the question of promotion is at issue!). In fact, at Leeds, we had only minimal support from the powers that be (for example in the 17 years I was there the department never boasted a technician), and I had the impression of working against rather than for the university. In more recent times, the syndrome is less surprising; similar situations seem to pervade the university world. Suffice it to say that for me, anyway, the writing was on the wall, and I spent my latter years at Leeds looking for a new position. In retrospect I feel myself fortunate that a number of positions for which I applied either wcre not offered to me or, on offer, I finally declined. In 1975 to my great surprise, I was approached about a position in The Netherlands, and in 1977 I was appointed professor of psychology in a fairly large Interfaculty of Physical Education (as it was then titled). The move was traumatic, the language even more so (master, teach thyself!), but all these traumata were offset by the working environment that I entered—good resources, technical support, and committed colleagues. Not to give a one-sided picture, I should indicate that there were many problems to be overcome before the faculty (some 10 years later) could achieve its present status of self-standing Faculty of Human Movement Sciences. But, I move ahead too quickly, and it is necessary to regress a little to my last years at Leeds.

Toward a Science of Human Movement

In the early 1970s my research interests began to extend not only within the field of skill acquisition but also into related fields like rehabilitation—notably that of motor impairment.

---

*In Dutch, *Enkel Reis* means a one-way trip.

A succession of advanced-diploma students contributed to my development in this latter area, culminating in 1971 in the publication of a review book on motor impairment written with one such student—Peter Morris (Morris & Whiting, 1971). This event was not only significant in its own right but it also reflected the status of my thinking at the meta level. In particular I was conscious of the limitation of the rubric *physical education* as an umbrella term for the kind of work in which we were involved.

This point of view became further enhanced following my move to the interfaculty in Amsterdam, because the concern there was not only with the study of human movement per se but more specifically with its relevance to people involved in the positive influencing of movement in professional fields as diverse as ergonomics, dance and the performing arts, education, sport, rehabilitation, and therapy. This kind of approach led me to the idea that as a consequence of the concern in these fields with the central concept of human movement, it might be useful to explore the possibility of a common body of knowledge on which all might draw. That body of knowledge I tentatively designated *human movement science*, recognizing with John Brooke (Brooke & Whiting, 1973) that

> men moving are multi-factorial organisms with such factors interacting with each other within the man, between men and in the relationships between men and their inanimate environment. Whatever position one adopts about the hierarchical ordering of these factors and their inter-relationships in determining the movement characteristics observed, it is clear that a network of interactions is being vitalized constantly and by such a process changing constantly. This poses problems for the scholar, who can no longer be restricted by the defined boundaries such as molecular biology, psychology, physiology, etc., within which to study separate aspects of human existence for they are not separate in this life situation. They participate together in the interacting systems of men and their environments, which systems neglect imposed divisions such as art-science, mind-body or social-individual dichotomies. (p. 3)

It seemed to me that a number of events—particularly in the prior 20 years—occurring in various parts of the world and at about the same time were forcing members of such professional fields as those listed previously to either supplement or in some cases replace their professional training, which had persisted in one form or another since the turn of the century and which in terms of academic content was often seriously deficient. This was not only a plea for so-called academic respectability—although that certainly played its part—but also a recognition of an issue to which Carr (1981) referred when he stated that "no . . . practice is theory or value free and if it doesn't follow from a body of coherent rationally informed judgments, then it will follow from a set of unreflectively common dogmas and prejudices" (p. 154).

In attempting to come to terms with this issue, professional institutions wishing to provide academic support for their professional activities had to either *develop* or *assemble* (and I use these words deliberately and distinctively) a body of relevant knowledge. It is perhaps not too surprising that differences of opinion should exist about the content of such a body of knowledge, the way in which it should be generated, and the name that it should be given.

What was often forgotten in this early enthusiasm for academic development—and is still forgotten at times—was that in order to meet the kind of professional developments being anticipated, such institutions must be professionally oriented. That is, their students must be equipped with a body of knowledge and a set of skills that enable the students, after a period of experience within a particular practical field, to address themselves effectively to the theoretical, practical, and research problems that arise in that field.

This plea for a particular attitude toward the study of human movement in faculties or institutions with a professional orientation is to be distinguished from the academic study of human movement per se. I addressed this issue in 1975 (Whiting, 1975b) when I expressed the opinion that human movement as a field of study is concerned with information that illuminates and integrates the diverse perspectives of the phenomenon of human movement. I deliberately did not include professional orientation in the discussion. Contributions to such a field of study were being made from disciplines as diverse as philosophy, cultural anthropology, neuropsychology, and biomechanics, to mention but a few. Many of the contributors to the development of a body of knowledge about human movement were only interested in the academic consequences of their work and not in its professional implications. In this sense, there has to be a difference between the orientations of such people with respect to the study of human movement and the orientations of people studying in the professional fields outlined. As I suggested in an earlier statement (Whiting, 1975b) "there is nothing implicit in the field of Human Movement Studies as I see it, to suggest a *necessary* link with . . . any . . . particular area of professional orientation which utilizes movement forms" (p. 2).

The study of human movement can be carried out purely for intrinsic and/or academic reasons in which a consideration of its relationship to any professional sphere of operation does not arise. In this sense, human movement studies are characterized—as indeed Renshaw (1975) proposed—simply by concern with the phenomenon of human movement. This definition acknowledges the importance of and contribution to be made by such disciplines as philosophy and the biological, physical, and social sciences.

To my mind, and in contrast to such an approach, any professional activity that is addressed to the positive influencing of human movement must be underpinned by an academic study of human movement—its focal point—a study that is relevant to the problems likely to arise in the field of concern. If this statement is accepted, we must then return to the essential question of how such a body of knowledge is assembled and developed.

The answer for any new field of academic study is relatively simple: A body of knowledge must be gleaned from the relevant parent disciplines. This makes some sense in the short term, because it is clear that a considerable amount of information about human movement—albeit mostly from a peripheral level of focus—is already available from within such disciplines and will continue to be generated, although this alone is unlikely to meet the ultimate needs of a professionally oriented faculty/ institution. In the long term, continued reliance on such sources of information alone can be both restrictive and misleading in that these sources are generally conceived in another context and may, in consequence, be less relevant or even irrelevant. What needs to be strived for is a particular form of what Wilberg (1972) termed "generated knowledge," that is, knowledge that arises from research involving problems in fields of professional operation that focus on the influencing of human movement.

Although this generated-knowledge idea is not new, it is often, with skilled argument, glossed over. For example, Broadbent (1971) addressed the problem in the context of pure and applied research. He made the point that the main issue is not necessarily the immediate economic importance of a piece of applied research, but rather that the problem is drawn from real life. By analogy, to generate a body of knowledge that is meaningful within the framework of human movement science, it is necessary to generate knowledge within the context of problems that arise, or might arise, within the many fields of professional application.

At the same time, we must recognize the multifaceted nature of such problems. For example, a patient undergoing rehabilitation may simultaneously present neurological, emotional, social, diagnostic, and re-educational problems. The specialized approach and data from one narrow discipline alone may be entirely inadequate for the best treatment of such a case. At some stage, a multidisciplinary approach needs to be taken in order to facilitate the grasp of a particular problem area. I have used the term *multidisciplinary* deliberately because however desirable an interdisciplinary approach might be, I am not sure at this stage of development of the field what this would imply or how it might be used.

In summary, the common body of knowledge with which students in the professional fields concerned with the influencing of human movement are confronted arises from a more comprehensive field of knowledge concerning what might be termed the human movement sciences. Further, selection from such a knowledge base must be made in terms of its relevance for such practical fields of operation. Although many of these fields, in terms of academic basis, are in early stages, selection from such a knowledge base may necessitate an undue reliance on recipient knowledge of a monodisciplinary nature; ultimately it must comprise knowledge generated from a multidisciplinary approach to problems arising directly from those fields of concern. Insofar as multidisciplinary study is reliant on methods and concepts developed within mono-disciplinary approaches, the contribution from such sources is not to be undervalued. This striving toward what Bernstein (1967) referred to as the science of human movements is a long-term aim of the journal *Human Movement Science*, which I founded shortly after arriving in Amsterdam.

The Amsterdam Connection

I was not the only one who was looking for such a change in direction; it was being actively pursued by others—notably at the University of Waterloo in Ontario, Canada. What really attracted me to Amsterdam was not only the position per se but a similar mentality among a number of members of the faculty, which was evident in their research and teaching interests. I joined a moving stream, and I like to think that I added something to the rate of flow. Nevertheless, we still had to wait until September 1987 before the interfaculty became a self-standing Faculty of Human Movement Sciences: a faculty comprising 7 chairs (one unfilled), 5 departments (exercise physiology and health science, educational sciences, functional anatomy, theoretical and historical studies, and psychology), and some 700 students.

My own research was limited during the early years in Amsterdam. Not only was it necessary to build up a new department (of psychology) but also to make a contribution (also administrative) to the development of the faculty as a whole. My particular concern was how the field of human movement science might be fostered. This was not a question of imposing a particular line of development on existing staff members but of creating an atmosphere in which that development might take place: not a completely self-organizing system, but one requiring only a minimum of cognitive steering! Significant issues contributed to the nature of that steering. For reasons not quite clear to me, I had never been particularly attracted to traditional psychological approaches to motor skills—particularly narrow laboratory experimental approaches—and preferred always to set my own line forward. Fairly early in my career (in the 1960s) I was influenced by Gibson's (1966) views on perception, and this was reflected—albeit tenuously—in my book *Acquiring Ball Skill: A Psychological Interpretation* (Whiting, 1969). In the early 1970s I also fell under the spells of the Russian physiologist Bernstein (1967) and the French phenomenologist Ricoeur (1966).

A succession of master's degree students at Leeds can attest to the seminar time spent on these two seminal texts. These lines of thinking carried over to Amsterdam, and although only recently made more explicit, they were a strong background influence on my department members. Just before leaving Leeds (1977) I conceived the idea of re-publishing Bernstein's (1967) book *The Coordination and Regulation of Movements* with commentary chapters from experts in the field of the human movement sciences, but I had to wait until 1984 (Whiting, 1984) before I could achieve that ambition. Again, in retrospect, the delay was worthwhile; the field expanded dramatically in the interim period.

It is not particularly interesting to catalog the course of events that led to the present situation in Amsterdam. Suffice it to say that in The Netherlands, around 1984, universities became caught up in what has been termed "conditional financing of research," which in essence necessitates that faculties establish coherent research programs (comprising subprograms that in turn comprise projects) involving a minimum of five full-time equivalent research positions. It quickly became clear that this was no choice situation but a matter of survival. Such programs had to receive positive appraisal both within the university as well as by externally established research bodies, future funding being dependent upon such appraisal. The psychology department of which I was chair received approval for its program on complex human motor actions (comprising the subprograms of acquisition of skill, training of motor skills, evaluation of movement patterns, and individual differences) in 1985. What is most significant, in the current context, is that in 1987 (following cooperative work with the Department of Theoretical and Historical Studies in our own faculty) we added an additional subprogram—conceptualizing human motor actions: the motor systems-action systems controversy. Thus, the intuitive feeling I had many years ago about the traditional field of motor skill became operationalized in the controversy.

In developing this latter metalevel subprogram, we found that we needed to develop a project area specifically directed to nonlinear dynamics and that this in itself implied a reorientation of departmental members—myself included—in a field of study for which their earlier training had ill-equipped them. Thus, in the twilight of my career I find myself having to return to the lecture room as student once again, this time in the knowledge that I am never going to graduate! But the trip will be worthwhile and younger staff members will complete it—isn't that what science is all about?

Part III

Autobiographies in Motor Development

Motor development is a specialized field of human action research concerned with describing and understanding the origins, development, and changes in human movement across the life span. As such, the field is concerned with understanding

- normal, universal changes arising out of the interaction of biological maturity and environmental influences (such as the normal locomotory transitions from crawling through upright stance to walking and running),
- individual differences in the rate of development of specific skills (e.g., motor performance comparisons between early and late developers),
- intertask differences in developmental competence, and
- the extreme deviancy from normative motor development evident among special populations (Connolly, 1986).

In its broadest context, motor development extends its concerns to not only the attainment of adult levels of motor performance by children but also to the gerontological issues associated with skill deterioration in the elderly. As we are faced with aging populations globally, research interest in the latter focus is bound to intensify in the coming decades.

The practical and theoretical importance of knowledge on motor development is substantial. Among other things, motor development knowledge is important practically for assessing the normative development of children in terms of their achievement of significant "motor milestones"; for providing understanding of the mechanisms of movement disabilities of all types and insight into how remedial and therapeutic programs might be most effectively structured; for ascertaining the readiness of individual learners for new skill acquisition tasks; and for providing a screening framework not only for the detection of movement disorders but also for the identification and nurturance of exceptional talent. Theoretically, motor development provides a critical testing ground for the efficacy both of general theories of development (predominantly arising from experimental psychology) and general theories of motor learning and control. The dependence on theoretical developments from these allied fields gives motor development questionable status as an independent subdiscipline of academic study. It is not clear whether motor development should be viewed as a specific element of the total field of development (e.g., see Smoll, 1982) or rather as an area of focus within the motor learning and control field (e.g., see J.R. Thomas & Thomas, 1989).

The history of motor development research reveals two quite disparate research approaches that vary in both the issues addressed and the methods and levels of analysis used (Wade, 1976). The oldest approach involves describing the critical "ages and stages" involved in the attainment of adult levels of performance of various fundamental motor skills (e.g., walking, running, jumping, and throwing). Concern is largely directed at determining when motor milestones for normative development are achieved. The second, more contemporary approach, involves attempting to explain how humans achieve given levels of motor performance at particular ages throughout the life span; this approach involves an attempt to experimentally ascertain the changes in the underlying control processes that accompany alterations in the maturational and experiential status of the performer. Such a focus brings the concerns of motor development very much in line with those of motor learning and control, to the point where *developmental motor learning* has been suggested as a more appropriate label for the modern field (Wade, 1976). Although the distinction between the descriptive, task-oriented approach and the explanation-seeking, process-oriented approach is common and widely accepted, the two approaches are not mutually exclusive. Description and explanation at a number of different levels are necessarily linked and complementary concerns for any science (see Keogh & Sugden, 1985; Rarick, 1982, chapter 7 of this book).

The descriptive approach has its origins in observational works of the 1920s and 1930s that chronicled developmental sequences in principally prehensive and locomotory tasks (e.g., Ames, 1937; Bayley, 1935; Burnside, 1927; Halverson, 1931; McCaskill & Wellman, 1938). These isolated research endeavors were replaced, beginning in the early 1940s, by a number of longitudinal research programs, some of which are still operative today. Notable large-scale endeavors include the University of California's Adolescent Growth Study (Espenschade, 1940; H.E. Jones, 1949); the University of Oregon's Medford Boys Growth Study (Clarke, 1971); the motor performance project initiated by Lawrence Rarick at the University of Wisconsin-Madison (see Rarick, chapter 7) and continued by Halverson and Roberton (Roberton, 1982); the Michigan State University project

(Seefeldt & Haubenstricker, 1982); and the University of Saskatchewan's Child Growth and Development Study (see Carron, chapter 10). The emergence of these programs of research, along with the appearance of Gesell and Ilg's (1946) influential but general developmental text, *The Child From Five to Ten*, is frequently taken as the formal identifiable beginnings of a motor development research field (Park, 1981). These early descriptive data were later fitted to general theories of cognitive intellectual development (e.g., Piaget, 1952) and to biological/genetical theories of development (e.g., Gesell, 1946). Data collection typically preceded theorizing (what we have labeled bottom-up experimentation), and theories that were used were imported from other fields rather than developed within the motor development field. The normative, descriptive approach to motor development dominated the field until the 1970s, focusing attention not only on the chronological development of fundamental motor skills (see Roberton, 1978, 1982 for reviews) but also on issues related to the relationship of motor performance to growth and development in all biological systems (e.g., Malina, 1979, 1981); the determination of essential motor abilities (e.g., Rarick, Dobbins, & Broadhead, 1976) and their linkage to intellectual development (e.g., Ismail, Kane, & Kirkendall, 1969); and individual (e.g., Rarick & Smoll, 1967) and sex (e.g., H.E. Jones, 1949; Rarick, 1961) differences in motor performance.

The field's transition to an explanation-seeking, process-oriented approach occurred in the early 1970s and was largely a response to a perceived lack of explanatory power within the existing literature and to the emerging popularity of the ubiquitous information-processing concept both in motor learning and control and in cognitive and developmental psychology. Connolly's (1970a) *Mechanisms of Motor Skill Development*, which was the edited proceedings of a 1968 London conference of the Centre for Advanced Study in the Developmental Sciences (CASDS), was a landmark for this transition in the approach to motor development research, although similar changes were also evident at the time in developmental psychology (e.g., Kendler, 1981, p. 325) and in ethology (Fentress, 1976). The adoption of the information-processing model as the theoretical framework for experimentation in motor development brought the investigative direction of motor development research in line with that of motor learning and control, albeit with some inevitable lag associated with the motor development field's paradigmatic dependence on the theoretical leads provided in the motor learning and control literature. Motor development research in the 1970s and early 1980s was characterized by the adoption of existing adult tests of information-processing stages to children of different ages. For example, researchers documented children's choice reaction time (e.g., Connolly, 1970b), reciprocal movement time (e.g., Sugden, 1980b), coincidence timing (e.g., Dorfman, 1977), and motor short-term memory (e.g., Winther & Thomas, 1981) using tests previously developed in the motor learning and control field to quantify the information-processing capacities and limitations of adults (see Gallagher, 1984; Keogh, 1981; Keogh & Sugden, 1985; J.R. Thomas, 1980 for reviews of this literature). Such experimentation was based on the now-questioned assumption that the processing stages underlying adult and child motor performance were identical and that the child was simply a poorer or less sophisticated information processor than the adult. The conclusion that emerged from much of this research was that the child appears to have access to processing capacities and resources ("hardware") that are comparable to those of the adult, but the child's performance is limited by his or her inefficient use of control strategies ("software") (Newell & Barclay, 1982). When subjects are provided appropriate strategies, many of the adult-child differences in performance can apparently be reduced or even eliminated (see Thomas, chapter 9).

The dynamical models that have risen to challenge the information-processing approach in motor learning and control made their initial appearances in the motor development field in Kelso and Clark's (1982) *The Development of Movement Control and Co-ordination*, an edited work arising from a conference held at the University of Iowa in 1980. In particular, the paper by Kugler, Kelso, and Turvey (1982) within this book still stands as a landmark presentation of the dynamical approach. By the time of the 1985 NATO Advanced Study Institute on Motor Skill Acquisition in Children held in Maastricht, The Netherlands (Wade & Whiting, 1986; Whiting & Wade, 1986), the dynamical/ecological model had generated a considerable following, and a special issue on motor development in *Developmental Psychology* (November, 1989) clearly reflected the continued emergence of this view. The work of Ester Thelen on the development of infant stepping and walking (e.g., Thelen, 1985, 1986, 1989; Thelen, Skala, & Kelso, 1987) provides perhaps the best example of a program of motor development research based on the dynamical model of motor control, whereas Mary Ann Roberton's work on relative timing in gait (Roberton, 1986) provides a clear example of how the emergence of the dynamical approaches has influenced the interpreting of data first collected with an information-processing perspective. The influence of the dynamical approach illustrates how the face of motor development research increasingly reflects shared interests with the motor learning and control field. The motor development field is currently grappling with the same methodological concerns related to the need for ecological validity and for process, as well as product, measures of motor performance evident in the motor learning and control field. Motor development has, in addition, some of its own unique, long-standing methodological concerns related to longitudinal versus cross-sectional, and idiographic versus nomethetic, research designs.

Our four contributors in this section have all played major roles in the historical and contemporary development of motor development research. Lawrence Rarick is undoubtedly the preeminent researcher associated with the normative, descriptive approach to motor development. Jack Keogh and David Sugden have been major contributors to the information-processing approach to motor development research, contributing especially to the isolation of information-processing capacities and limitations, not only in children without disabilities, but also in children drawn from special populations. Their two joint texts (Keogh & Sugden, 1985; Sugden & Keogh, 1990) are the definitive works in regard to motor development in both normal and special populations. Jerry Thomas has also contributed heavily to process-oriented inquiry in motor development although from more varied perspectives than Keogh and Sugden. He has been involved in the testing, in the motor development context, of neo-Piagetian theories and classical information-processing notions (especially related to strategy utilization); more recently, he has been a prime mover in applying the expert-novice paradigm to the development of sport skills. His recent concern with the biomechanics of gender differences in throwing reflects an emerging interest in the dynamics of developing movement control.

Chapter 6

Jack F. Keogh

Department of Kinesiology
University of California at Los Angeles
Los Angeles, California, U.S.A.

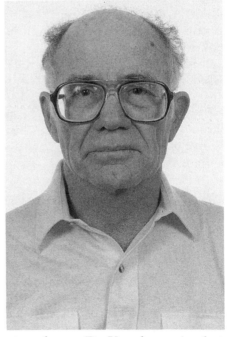

J ack Keogh completed a bachelor of arts degree at Pomona College in 1949 and an MS degree at Claremont Graduate School in 1951, and he spent over 6 years as a physical education instructor in a range of high school and junior college settings before commencing his doctoral studies at the University of California, Los Angeles (UCLA) in 1956. He was awarded an EdD in 1959 after completing his doctoral studies in concert with work as a teaching assistant at UCLA (1956-57) and as an instructor at Pomona College (1957-59). Immediately upon his graduation he joined the faculty of what was then the Department of Physical Education at UCLA as an assistant professor. Dr. Keogh remained at UCLA until he retired in 1987 as a full professor within the Department of Kinesiology. During his tenure at UCLA Professor Keogh served as departmental chair (1974-77) and as director of the Bureau of Education for the Handicapped's Graduate Research Training Project (1971-82). As his autobiographical chapter reveals, a sabbatical leave spent from 1965 to 1966 as a postdoctoral fellow at the University of Birmingham in

England served as an important stimulus for his lasting research contribution to the motor development field.

The transitions within Jack Keogh's personal career bear strong parallels to the history of the motor development field. In his early research work (much of which is summarized in Keogh & Sugden, 1985) he collected normative data on motor performance using longitudinal data collection methods and samples of elementary school children with no apparent disabilities. His focus then shifted to the question of movement disorders among special populations (especially those with learning and intellectual disorders). Keogh's most significant change in focus, and in turn his most significant contribution to the motor development field, has been his identification of the problems of motor development as problems of movement control; this identification has concomitant implications for the need to observe and measure process variables in addition to making simple performance (product) measures. In this respect, his 1977 *Quest* paper remains among his most influential, although his two texts with David Sugden on the motor development of nondisabled populations (Keogh & Sugden, 1985) and special populations (Sugden & Keogh, 1990) are his most comprehensive and will undoubtedly be his most broadly influential. Keogh has also published extensively in the movement confidence area (e.g., Griffin & Keogh, 1982; Keogh, Griffin, & Spector, 1981), rekindling an early interest in personality research. He has served the discipline through stints on the editorial boards of the *Research Quarterly for Exercise and Sport* and *Exercise and Sport Sciences Reviews*, as well as serving at various times as a consulting reviewer/adviser for the *American Journal of Mental Deficiency, Child Development*, and the *Journal of Psychoeducational Assessment*.

Jack Keogh's autobiographical chapter chronicles clearly the thinking that underlies changes in approach and focus that have characterized not only his own career but the motor development field in general. His emphasis on the need for measurement of movement process in addition to measurement of outcome is topical for all experimenters in motor learning and control as well as motor development, although his use of qualitative, observational methods in addition to quantitative measures makes his approach somewhat unique. The research style he describes in this chapter is predominantly problem .and data driven, emphasizing breadth of knowledge as essential for the ultimate progression of the field. Note in particular his observation that a number of the conceptual breakthroughs that were, at the time, major revelations for motor development research are with the benefit of retrospection embarrassingly obvious. As Scott Kelso also noted in his chapter, clarity after a discovery has been made appears to be the norm for almost all scientific developments of substance.

AUTOBIOGRAPHY

My professional involvement in physical activity started in a way common to others—by teaching physical education and coaching athletic teams, particularly ball games in which team play was important. Skill intrigued me in terms of how an individual could move in so many elegant ways and how personality, as it then was labeled, seemed so important in the effective use of skill with other participants in relation to rapidly changing events. My formal academic involvement started in 1956, when I was a graduate student with the modest goal of understanding everything about movement skill and personality of elite performers. Several years of musings led me to study movement skill development in a way that has taken me across a broad terrain rather than into the depths of a region, which is the more common approach after one learns that there are limits to what one can know and comprehend.

The lack of theories and models in movement development accounts for part of my wanderings as a search process, but an equal part resides in my love of wondering and wandering. No single study is critical in relating my intellectual travels to acquire my assorted views about movement skill development, which are stated in two books (Keogh & Sugden, 1985; Sugden & Keogh, 1990) that represent 30 years of academic involvement. What I wish to describe here is a major change in my thinking about movement skill development that occurred in the middle to late 1960s.

Personality of elite performers quickly lost its charm for me, probably when I recognized that I was more interested in less skilled persons who found great satisfaction in movement activities. My focus shifted to participation in terms of what gets a person involved, what influences his or her effort, and what are important personal satisfactions. Attitude seemed like a possible key to understanding participation, but I was not comfortable with attitude measurements and related analyses. Also, I realized that I wanted to understand how all of this came to be, which meant studying children. This general metamorphosis in my thinking took several years. I dropped my work on personality and attitude to focus on development of movement skill as a more manageable area of study and one that fit my research abilities. My plan at that time was to return later to personal aspects of participation that could be studied in relation to movement skill development, which I did briefly in studying movement confidence (Griffin & Keogh, 1982; Griffin, Keogh, & Maybee, 1984).

Movement skill development, as an area of study, was in the doldrums in the early 1960s when I decided this was the place for me. Earlier descriptive studies provided normative data for medical personnel and psychologists interested in early development and for educators interested in play-game performance of school children. Some work was being done to relate physical growth characteristics and movement capabilities, but the movement measures were limited in scope in terms of being strength oriented, involving topics such as maximal efforts to jump and throw. Some careful biomechanical analyses of specific movements were being made, although not in a way that would help us understand skill development beyond the task being analyzed. Generally, there was very little in the way of systematic programs of research. Given this state of the art, it was no wonder that there were no models or theories of movement skill development being pursued. The field was wide open and I was drawn to this openness.

I decided to focus on ages 3 to 10, because play-game skills are developed and refined during these years. Children in this age range are beyond the more fundamental development of postural control, locomotion, and manual movements but are not yet confounded with pubertal development, except for early maturing girls. I also was and still am impressed with cognitive and personal-social changes during these years that need to be studied in relation to movement skill development. My next problem was where to begin in terms of studying movement skill changes. Given the lack of useful frameworks or structures with which to conceptualize skill changes during these years, I decided that my first step was to gather a considerable volume of skill performance data, including longitudinal measures, which would provide me with a basis for thinking about movement skill development. That is, I needed to do some looking on my own as a way to get beyond group mean data so that I could formulate ideas to be tested.

I initiated a project in 1963 to test play-game skills of elementary school children (ages 5 to 12) in Santa Monica, California. I took considerable care with methodological details, because I needed the best data possible for my study of movement skill development and I felt that much of the existing normative data was seriously flawed. As a simple example, we grouped boys and girls by age rather than by grade level, because some children were as much as 1 year older or younger than their classmates.

The important part of the project was a longitudinal study of 6-year-olds and 8-year-olds who were tested twice per year for 4 years. We observed individual change and kept observational notes of performance to provide additional information for me to ponder. Our observations were focused on inadequate and "almost" performances of children. My general logic was (and now is) that the time to study development is when a skill is emerging or is changing markedly, rather than when a skill is being refined to produce a maximal achievement. The normative results and longitudinal analyses of this 4-year project were placed in two technical reports for the granting agency (Keogh, 1965, 1969) and later were summarized briefly in the first book (Keogh & Sugden, 1985).

During these years the perceptual-motor craze was sweeping the country. Children with learning problems, which included everything from severe mental retardation to specific reading problems, were receiving an unusual amount of professional and public attention. Numerous theories and interventions were proposed in which perceptual-motor problems and related instructional procedures were key features. The main thrust of this thinking was that movement is important in perceptual development and thus is important in remediation of perceptual problems that were presumed to be underlying causes in cognitive problems. The focus, therefore, was on the impact of movement on perception, and there was little concern for the impact of perceptual development on movement development (Keogh, 1978). I received many inquiries from those involved in perceptual-motor training programs because I was studying movement skill development, even though I had little knowledge of classroom learning problems. This led me to become involved in instructional programs for children with movement skill problems, which is merely another kind of learning problem (Keogh, 1982).

The major event in my story began with an invitation from the Kennedy Foundation to be a consultant for a summer physical activity program for children with mental retardation, held at the Shriver estate in Bethesda, Maryland. A second consultant, whom I had not met before, was James Oliver from Birmingham University in England. Following 2 weeks of intense interaction with Oliver in June 1964, I returned to Los Angeles knowing that I wanted to work with him during my sabbatical leave in 1965-66. I was able to do this, with financial support provided by the newly formed National Institute of Child Health and Human Development. This year of work with Oliver led to a major change in my thinking about movement skill development.

The formal purpose of my study leave was to study movement skill performance of children with mental retardation, but a personal goal was to learn more of what Oliver knew about movement skill problems. I particularly wanted to observe him working with individual children. Like most gifted teachers, he was adept at getting a child involved and in analyzing the child's skill problems. Even more impressive was his ability to articulate what he was thinking and then show me how he tested the problem possibilities by restructuring the assessment and instructional environment. Beyond doing several formal studies, I spent my time finding children with movement skill problems and observing Oliver work individually with these children. As the year passed, we spent more time discussing general issues related to movement, skill, and development; the movement skill problems of individual children provided illustrations or data to make or test a point.

A major change in my thinking emerged from this year of study away from my home base in the company of a colleague who knowingly and unknowingly introduced me to new ideas and concepts. I came to view development of movement skill as the change from lack of control to achievement of basic control (Keogh, 1971). Achieving upright locomotion (walking), reaching to touch an object, and performing thumb-finger opposition (neat pincer grasp) are classic illustrations of achieving basic control during early months after birth. Subsequent achievements build upon achievements such as these, so that it is difficult after the early months of a subject's development to study the change from lack of control to achievement of basic control. However, it is important that we think about development as change in control rather than measure and analyze skill changes in terms of maximal performance scores or efficient mechanics.

As I reflect on my experiences, I find that my thinking changed because I became involved in observing and thinking about children with movement skill problems. Traditional evaluations were done in terms of normative expectations, which were primarily scores that indicated how many, how far, how fast, and how often. I soon found that Oliver watched how children did whatever they did. He noticed that a boy who was mentally retarded could not skip because he could not hop on his right foot. Oliver worked with the boy for several minutes twice in one day to get him hopping on his right foot and to help him alternate leg movements. Early the next morning, the boy skipped haltingly but wildly around the playground to show us his newly found skill, which he had practiced for hours after leaving us the previous day. We next saw him weeks later when he demonstrated a versatile array of skipping skills that included going in circles with his arms alternately pumping up and down as if he were doing a tribal dance. The change in this movement skill and the enthusiastic behavior of the child reminded me that these were the two halves of the world I someday hoped to understand.

Oliver's simple observations of movement mechanics provided a basis for analysis of movement skill problems and led to instructional applications. These observations had long-term value for me because they forced my attention toward what might be limiting a child's achievement of basic control of a movement skill that much younger children were capable of achieving. For example, some children seemed to lack postural control adequate to stabilize the body when running fast, whereas others could not time their arms and hands to meet a moving ball. The same observations must be true for normal development of a movement skill, except these or similar problems occur at an earlier age.

All of this led me to realize that the movement skill problems I was observing were manifestations of whatever were the controlling systems. In a simplified sense, movement is the product of the functioning of the neuromotor system, as serviced by other physiological systems, in coordination with perceptual-cognitive information to specify internal and external conditions, make action decisions, and monitor situation outcomes. This revelation will seem embarrassingly naive to those who entered the field in subsequent years, but the study of movement development at this time was linked to medical and educational assessment and intervention and was not concerned with how movement was produced. The study of movement skill of adults focused primarily on performance enhancement related to specific types of achievements such as operating machines, flying airplanes, and participating in sports. It was several years before some of the researchers studying movement performance and learning became concerned with how movements were controlled, which now is a major line of inquiry.

I returned from England with my thinking thoroughly disrupted, but I was excited about the idea of control. My immediate problem was that I knew I needed to change radically the focus of my work, but I did not know where to begin. I followed the path of least resistance by continuing my observations of movement skill performance of children with an eye to formulating general impressions and ideas about development of movement control. This meant that I must find movements to observe that would help me view changes in movement control. This was not easy, because most movement tasks in use at that time were used to test the subject's ability to generate maximal force and/or speed. Also, I did not yet want to include movements involving spatial-temporal responses to a changing or unstable environment. My work with Oliver led me to think about limb movements, because he placed great emphasis on watching the limbs. His rationale was simply that limb movements are needed to create and alter most body movements. Observing the control of limb movements thus became my way of observing development of movement control.

I did considerable preliminary work to select a set of movement tasks. The limb movements had to be self-paced, as well as continuous with an overall rhythm, and could not require maximal force and maximal speed. Examples are alternate tapping of pencils that the individual holds in each hand, alternate tapping of feet while the individual is sitting, and movement of feet out to the side and back to the midline while the subject is standing.

The performance score was merely pass or fail; to pass, the individual had to perform five continuous repetitions of the basic movement cycle. However, the behavior I wanted to watch went beyond pass or fail. My problem was what to watch and how to measure it. For example, many boys made forceful and almost discrete limb movements. They alternated pencil taps with forceful, full arm movements and followed each hand movement with their eyes. Most girls had easy wrist motions, seldom watched their movements, and sometimes even talked to the examiner as if the tapping movements were automatic or at least did not require much attention. I knew that movement differences of this nature were what I needed to observe, because they helped me conceptualize movement skill development as changes in movement control of parameters such as changes in force modulation, joint actions, and attentional requirements. Some of these movement differences can be seen in biomechanical measures, whereas others, such as attentional requirements, must be inferred from observed behaviors.

After I experienced much frustration in trying to create measures for the many things I now viewed as part of movement control, I finally realized that I was ahead of the game and did not need a formal set of measurements at this time. What I needed were more observations of children's movements, as I had made with Oliver, observations made in the way that one might watch children solve puzzles to note the variety and richness of the children's strategies. As I noted something that seemed important, such as force modulation and attentional requirements, I then changed requirements in tasks currently in my repertoire or devised a new limb movement task to observe how children solved the new problem. I was using somewhat natural observations to see how children did what they did, and I concentrated on what I could infer about their development of movement control.

I spent several years observing limb movement tasks, during which time I completed a project that indicated children improve in performance during ages 5 to 9, with striking differences in favor of girls. The age and sex comparisons were based on both pass/fail percentages and observational data about qualitative differences (Keogh, 1968). Although this project has not impacted the field in any way that I know, it was my most important work in terms of formulating my perspective about movement skill development.

My comments thus far have been primarily about movement and skill, but the most important outcome of my focusing on control was the way it directed my thinking about development. It forced me to recognize that development was more than bigger and better. Given that development is change, I needed to know the nature of the many changes that provide our descriptive sense of development. As noted earlier, I reasoned that movement skill is produced primarily by neuromotor and perceptual-cognitive systems. Development, therefore, must be a function of changes in these systems, which I identify as a function of changes in personal resources. This means that the study of movement skill development involves the study of development of personal resources in relation to changes in movement skills.

Environmental conditions and task requirements are the features in a particular movement situation that are common to each mover. As level of development of personal resources increases, movement skill increases in relation to the same environmental conditions and task requirements. That is, a child's proficiency in using a spoon to get cereal from a bowl into his or her mouth progresses from holding the spoon in a fixed grasp with no wrist movement (which precludes adjustment of the spoon) to a manipulation of spoon position by use of finger and wrist movement. The child also progresses to a dual-task achievement of listening to others while using the spoon.

It is important that the researcher note carefully the environmental conditions and task requirements that define the movement problem to be resolved, but the study of movement skill development must also focus on the changes in personal resources that make it possible for a subject to deal with different types of movement problems. I drafted a book in 1971 in an effort to use this general perspective as a structure for organizing existing descriptive data. After consultation with two helpful editors, I decided that the book was premature because there were too many holes in my thinking and in what I knew about several key topics. I wrote the book 10 years later in partnership with David Sugden, another Englishman who helped me clarify the general structure and who added knowledge in areas that were beyond my ken (Keogh & Sugden, 1985). We followed with a second book to review movement skill problems of children with major deficiencies in personal resources, including cerebral palsy, blindness, and mental retardation, in an effort to learn what these conditions might teach us about movement skill development (Sugden & Keogh, 1990).

More than 20 years have passed since my academic happening that began with my interactions with Oliver and led to my observations of limb movements. This change in my thinking has primarily affected my further thinking about movement, skill, and development, rather than affecting my methods of testing particular ideas. Weiss (1969) noted that scientists too often stay buried in their particular burrows and need occasionally to reflect on where they are headed and how their problems fit into a larger scene, as prairie dogs might put their heads out of the burrow to see where they are. I have worked in a different way by wandering across the terrain to seek a broader sense of what is involved in movement skill development with only an occasional bit of burrowing before I once again emerge to travel some more. As a concluding comment, I want to note a general change I have observed in the landscape during the past 20 years.

Publication of *Mechanisms of Motor Skill Development* (Connolly, 1970a) was exciting for me and my students, because the book pointed to the study of movement control in relation to the development of personal resources. Both the beauty and the beast of this book were that the conference contributors were established scientists in fields not directly involved in studying movement. The book discussed new issues and questions that should have led to changes in thinking about movement skill development. The eventual drawback was that movement skill development was a secondary and not a continuing focus for most of the contributors. There was stimulation for the field of movement development but few were ready at that time to extend these ideas.

Themes in Motor Development, an edited volume by Whiting and Wade (1986), provides a measure of progress since 1970. The contributors again were established scientists, but some were from the fields of physical education and kinesiology. More importantly, movement skill development was the primary study interest for many of the conference participants. I see that the study of movement skill development has emerged from the doldrums of several decades past with an influx of scientists trained in other fields or in other aspects of movement and skill who are using models and theories to direct their work.

Chapter 7

G. Lawrence Rarick

Department of Physical Education
University of California at Berkeley
Berkeley, California, U.S.A.

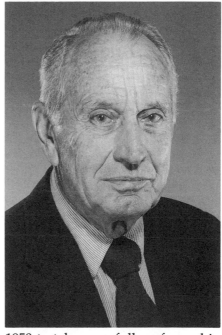

P rior to and while teaching in a junior-senior high school in Ransom, Kansas, Lawrence Rarick completed AB, BS, and MS degrees at Fort Hays Kansas State College, presently Fort Hays Kansas State University (in 1933, 1933, and 1935, respectively). He followed these degrees with a PhD in physical education from the State University of Iowa in 1937 under the joint tutelage of C.H. McCloy and W.W. Tuttle. Upon completing his doctorate, Rarick held teaching positions at the University of Wichita from 1937 to 1941 and, from 1941 to 1950, at Boston University (excluding a 2-1/2-year period of service in the U.S. Naval Reserve). He moved to Madison in 1950 to take up a full professorship in physical education at the University of Wisconsin, where he remained until moving to the Department of Physical Education at the University of California at Berkeley in 1968. Dr. Rarick became professor emeritus at the University of California, Berkeley, in 1979, nevertheless retaining an active research interest and publication profile in motor development throughout the 1980s.

Rarick's role in the formation of motor development as a credible field of academic research is without parallel. He has influenced the direction of the motor development field through intensive and extensive personal research activity and productivity, through the initiation of major longitudinal research programs both at the University of Wisconsin and at Berkeley, and through the training of graduate students (such as Robert Malina) who in turn have greatly influenced contemporary growth and development research. Like Franklin Henry and John Whiting in the motor learning and control field, Rarick has maintained a concern not only for his specialized field but also for the broader discipline of physical education research, a discipline that he profoundly influenced through important contributions to the debates on the philosophical nature of disciplinary study in physical education/kinesiology (e.g., Rarick, 1967).

Professor Rarick has also contributed to the discipline through editorial work for *Medicine and Science in Sports, Research Quarterly, Journal of Motor Behavior,* and *Adapted Physical Activity Quarterly.* His contribution to the motor development field and to physical education in general has been rewarded by a number of honors and awards, including fellowship of the American Academy of Physical Education; the alliance scholar award of the American Alliance for Physical Education, Health, Recreation and Dance (for 1979-80); the distinguished scholar award of the North American Society for the Psychology of Sport and Physical Activity (NASPSPA; in 1981); and a tribute volume on the academic discipline of physical education (Brooks, 1981).

His research activity in motor development has arisen primarily from the large motor performance and anthropometric databases he collected as part of his numerous and ambitious longitudinal studies on boys and girls drawn from both disabled and nondisabled populations. What has resulted has been invaluable information on age, sex, and maturational differences in motor performance (e.g., Rarick & Oyster, 1964; Rarick & Thompson, 1956); information on motor abilities and their stabilities from early childhood to adolescence (e.g., Rarick & Smoll, 1967); descriptions of motor ability and performance deficits in children with Down syndrome (e.g., Rarick, Rapaport, & Seefeldt, 1966) and mental retardation (e.g., Rarick, Dobbins, & Broadhead, 1976); and experimental findings on the effectiveness of physical activity programs in aiding motor, cognitive, social, and emotional development of educationally disabled children (Rarick et al., 1976). His edited text from 1973, *Physical Activity: Human Growth and Development,* remains an enduring contribution to motor development in its broadest context.

Rarick's research work is characterized (as this chapter reveals) by data-driven or problem-driven experimentation, and he remains a staunch defender of the importance of descriptive non-theory-driven experimentation for the development of knowledge in all areas, including motor development (see also Rarick, 1982). His chapter shows a somewhat unique multidisciplinary orientation within his experimentation and a sophisticated use of complex data analytic methods. Note in reading his chapter how the factor analytic work within his doctoral studies on traits and abilities in athletic performance ideally prepared him to later apply innovative multivariate methods to the study of motor development. Also note how a number of chance external factors (and in particular, his initial teaching assignment at Boston University) were largely responsible for directing his career-long research endeavors to the problems posed by motor development.

AUTOBIOGRAPHY

Research careers are shaped by a multitude of interacting factors that are in most cases difficult to sort out. For some, the selection of a research career and the direction it takes are results of long-term planning, but I suspect that for most, this career choice is the result of changing circumstances over which the individual has limited control.

In reflecting on my own career of some 50 years, I clearly see that the direction my research has taken is more a function of the situations in which I found myself than it is of long-range planning. Although one might say opportunities are made by the individual, I suspect that most researchers will admit that being in the right place at the right time is of more than passing importance.

The Early Years

During my youth and undergraduate days I gave little thought to an academic-research career. Attending a small midwestern college during the Great Depression and having a long-time interest in sports, I prepared for a teaching-coaching career. Once embarked on this pursuit I saw it as a temporary undertaking. During the summer months I began graduate study in chemistry with the view of applying for admission to a medical school; I also considered the possibility of advanced study in a health-related field. Hence, I applied for admission both to a medical school and for graduate study in physical education. Both applications were acted on favorably, but sensing that by temperament I was ill-suited for a medical career, I accepted a scholarship for graduate study in physical education at the State University of Iowa. At that time doctoral study in physical education was offered in a limited number of universities. The department at Iowa, with a research-oriented faculty and its tie with the university medical school, was one of the top departments of that era.

The years at Iowa opened my eyes to the research opportunities in physical education. This was largely a reflection of the presence there of C.H. McCloy and W.W. Tuttle, who were at the peaks of their research productivity. I was fortunate to have them as joint advisers on my PhD research.

Near the start of my 2nd year at Iowa I selected a thesis topic that cut across physical education and exercise physiology, namely a problem that focused on the speed of muscular movement in humans. A.V. Hill (1927) had proposed some years earlier that the major factor limiting the velocity of muscle contraction is muscle viscosity, the internal passive resistance that opposes rapid change in the state of contracting muscle fibers. According to Hill (1927) the work done by a muscle in shortening can be expressed as a simple function of the velocity of contraction by the equation

$$W = Wo \ (1 - Kv)$$

where Wo represents the work a muscle can do under conditions of maximum effort when shortening infinitely slowly. If one gives the muscle a lighter load, allowing it to shorten with increasing velocity v, the work W accomplished becomes less than Wo, even though the muscle continues to exert maximum effort. Hill (1927) verified this equation with human arm muscle, a relationship that would hold were there an internal resistance of a viscous character. While holding to his viscosity theory, Hill (1927) did propose that an increase in propelling force might well be as effective in increasing velocity of muscle shortening as would occur with a lower velocity.

The research design that I employed (Rarick, 1937) followed Thurstone's (1935) concept that human traits are complex in nature and are made up of certain general abilities upon which the individual may draw as well as abilities that are specific to the task. In brief, I hypothesized that speed of movement in athletic activities conducted with maximum effort is a complex phenomenon drawing on such basic components as muscular strength and force, characteristics of the muscle tissue and its nerve supply, length of bony levers, body weight (negative factor), and possibly other factors and/or specifics. I selected some test items that would logically call primarily on one hypothesized factor and other test items that would in turn call on other factors, so each factor in the hypothesized factor structure was properly represented by test items.

I gave some 22 laboratory and field tests to 51 University of Iowa varsity athletes, intercorrelating the test results and factoring the intercorrelation matrix with Thurstone's (1935) method of multiple factors. The field tests were for the most part athletic tests requiring maximum propulsive force of the body as a whole or of its limbs. The laboratory tests included measures of dynamometric strength, reaction time, and muscle thickening latency (a measure of the time interval between electrical stimulation of the muscle's motor point and the first physical evidence of muscle contraction).

The resulting factor analysis isolated six factors, the most prominent a speed or velocity factor that was identified by the high loading of variables requiring explosive muscular force as in maximum effort of running, jumping, and throwing. Strength as assessed by tests of dynamometric strength of the arms, back, and legs emerged as a factor. The low loadings of these variables on the velocity factor provided evidence that static strength above a certain minimum contributed little to the speed of movement as assessed by the tests. The other factors such as length of bony levers, muscle thickening latency, and arm strength accounted for only a little of the variance, whereas, not surprisingly, body weight was a negative factor. Perhaps the most significant finding of the study was the limited importance of isometric strength in forceful rapid muscle contractions, a finding that was repeatedly verified by later investigations.

Following the completion of my dissertation I held successive appointments at the University of Wichita and at Boston University, interspersed with a period of military service during World War II. At Boston University one of my assignments was to teach a graduate-undergraduate course in child development and to guide the research of students with an interest in motor development, an assignment that changed the course of my professional career. When the opportunity came to go to the University of Wisconsin in 1950 with a primary responsibility for initiating a teaching and research program in motor development, I accepted the post.

The Wisconsin Years

Almost at the outset of my tenure at the University of Wisconsin, I embarked on a longitudinal study of the motor development of school-age children. The rationale for using the longitudinal approach was based on the premise that longitudinal data are necessary if one is interested in studying the individuality of growth curves, the stability and predictability of human characteristics, and the factors affecting developmental change. Prior to this, several large-scale longitudinal studies had been done on the physical growth of school-age children as well as studies of motor development in infancy, but few if any had dealt with motor development of children of elementary school age.

I knew full well the problems of longitudinal field studies, such as dropouts, test sensitization, motivational difficulties, provision for experimental controls, and obtaining an appropriate sample. In spite of this I felt that the advantages far outweighed the disadvantages, if proper precautions were taken. Furthermore, the longitudinal method provided me the opportunity to seek answers to questions about the motor behavior of children at various developmental stages without disturbing the major thrust of the research.

I obtained permission from school administrators and parents of children attending two suburban Madison elementary schools to embark on a longitudinal field study of physical growth and motor development commencing with 1st-grade boys and girls. The primary purpose of the investigation (Rarick & Smoll, 1967) was to observe annual changes in the gross motor performance (muscle strength, motor performance, and movement patterns) of boys and girls through the childhood years and into later adolescence, as well as to determine some of the factors that influenced these changes. This was a collaborative undertaking in that a colleague (Ruth Glassow) used cinematography to assess movement patterns of the children in running, jumping, and throwing, and I supervised the collection of the physical growth, strength, and motor performance data. The latter included 12 anthropometric measures; 10 measures of dynamometric strength; radiographic measures of bone, muscle, and subcutaneous tissue of the calf; and X rays of the hand and wrist, the latter for the assessment of bone age.

This extensive database provided me the opportunity to conduct a series of cross-sectional studies, only two of which will be mentioned here. The first (Rarick & Thompson, 1956) was designed to determine sex differences in the strength of young children after controlling for muscle mass as revealed from soft tissue radiographs. We used strength of the ankle extensors as the criterion measure, assuming that habitual use of the legs in locomotion by young children should not differ materially between the sexes.

The findings clearly showed that indeed males had significantly greater strength as early as age 7, even after we controlled for sex differences in muscle mass. The strength difference may have reflected sex differences in the quality of muscle tissues or perhaps motivational differences under the conditions of testing.

A second study (Rarick & Oyster, 1964) enabled us to determine the effect of physical maturity (as assessed by hand-wrist X rays) on the muscular strength and motor proficiency of young boys. In other words, was a measure of physical maturity as significant as chronological age, height, and weight in predicting muscle strength and motor performance of 8-year-old males? We used eight measures of muscle strength and three measures of motor performances and found by the use of partial and multiple correlations that bone age did not add significantly to age, height, and weight in the prediction of either strength or motor performance as assessed here.

The major thrust of the longitudinal investigation was examination of the stability of physical growth and motor performance over the childhood years and into adolescence. Early longitudinal studies (Shuttleworth, 1939; Tuddenham & Snyder, 1954) on physical growth indicated that both height and weight could be predicted with considerable accuracy from childhood to later adolescence. Our findings (Rarick & Smoll, 1967) on the physical growth measures agreed with the earlier reports. However, between year correlations (7-17 years) on the strength and motor performance measures were considerably lower. In the case of the strength measures, the majority of the correlations (7-17 years) were in the .30s and .40s with some in the .50s and .60s. These correlations compared favorably with those reported by Tuddenham and Snyder (1954) on grip and shoulder girdle strength of males over the age span 9 to 18 years. On the motor performance tests, half of the correlations were in the .50s or higher, the remainder being somewhat lower. Our findings clearly show that the prediction of motor performance from the early childhood years to later adolescence is hazardous.

During the early years of the longitudinal study, a colleague in the University of Wisconsin Department of Psychiatry, who had liaison with the Wisconsin state institutions for the mentally retarded, approached me about a collaborative longitudinal study that would use radiographic methods for studying physical maturity and growth of bone and soft tissues in children with Down syndrome. This initiated a 12-year study (Rarick, Rapaport, & Seefeldt, 1964, 1965, 1966), for which we took yearly radiographs (leg, hand, and wrist) on some 74 children with Down syndrome, the youngest age level initially being 6 years. This enabled us, among other things, to determine the age at which ossification centers of certain bones of the hand and wrist appear, the rate of development of these bones, the tempo of growth of bone and soft tissues in the calf, the time of epiphyseal fusion of the tibia, and the relationship of these events to the onset of puberty.

Space will permit only a few general comments on the findings. As one would expect, there was substantial delay in development of all measures, but as we observed the measures from year to year it became evident that the children with Down syndrome, although markedly behind the standards on nondisabled children, were nevertheless maintaining approximately the same tempo of growth as children who were not disabled. In other words, our data provided evidence that the retardation in growth came during the first 5 to 6 years of life; after that, the velocity of growth of the children with Down syndrome kept pace with that of their nondisabled counterparts. Furthermore, when we compared the growth curves of our sample of children with Down syndrome with a sample of nondisabled children using a double logistic model, we found that the circumpubertal growth curves of the two, although differing in magnitude, did not differ in form (Rarick, Wainer, Thissen, & Seefeldt, 1975). Similarly, the timing of epiphyseal fusion of the tibia in the boys and girls with Down syndrome was associated with the usual indicators of puberty in ways similar to that of nondisabled children (Rarick et al., 1966). Thus, our findings indicated that the biological forces that initiate and control growth during the circumpubertal years appear to function similarly in children with Down syndrome and those without.

Again, circumstance played a role in initiating my research on the motor domain of children who are mentally retarded. A departmental colleague at Wisconsin obtained funding, from what at the time was the Cooperative Research Branch of the U.S. Office of Education, to study the motor characteristics of children who are mentally retarded. After I helped him design motor tests appropriate for this project, he became ill and asked me to assume major responsibility for completing the project. This study (Francis & Rarick, 1959), although limited in scope (involving some 280 children in the schools of Milwaukee and Madison who were educable mentally retarded), did show that these children were, on the average, from 2 to 4 years behind the motor performance levels of nonretarded children of the same age. Sex differences in performance were approximately the same as those for nonretarded children, and the correlations of the test items with measures of intelligence were relatively low, similar to the correlations on nonretarded children.

In view of the small sample size of this study, I decided to seek funding for a similar study (Rarick, Widdop, & Broadhead, 1970) with nationwide scope. My colleagues and I obtained such funding from the Joseph P. Kennedy, Jr. Foundation. We drew a multistage probability sample of children aged 8-18 years from the educable mentally retarded classrooms in the contiguous states of the United States, limiting the sample size to approximately 4,000 children, some 200 of each sex at each age level. Before embarking on the testing program (AAHPER Youth Fitness Test), we conducted a pilot study in Madison, which resulted in minor modifications in certain test items. Trained testers traveled by plane or car to the locations of the 40 primary sampling units of 100 children each.

The results essentially supported the earlier findings of the Wisconsin sample, namely that the boys who were retarded were consistently 1 standard deviation (SD) below the mean of nonretarded boys on the test items, and the girls who were retarded were 1/2 to 1 SD below the mean of nonretarded girls. Norms for these children on each test item were established by sex for each age level and also according to an age-height-weight classification index. During this general time frame several reports (Corder, 1966; Nunley, 1965; Oliver, 1958) were published that indicated a positive influence of physical activity programs on the cognitive development of children who are educationally disabled. The rationales for the reported improvements were not clearly spelled out in these studies, and the research designs were in no sense flawless.

In view of these developments I sensed that the time was right for a major investigation that would circumvent many of the shortcomings of these earlier studies. Thus, upon completion of our national study, I drafted a proposal for funding of a study that employed a multivariate design appropriate for assessing the effects of school physical activity programs on selected measures of the motor, cognitive, social, and emotional development of children who were educationally disabled. It was important that such a study be conducted in a reasonably typical public school setting, that it extend for a sufficient period of time to permit the experimental program to be put to the test, that the measures employed have acceptable validity, that proper experimental controls be used, and that teachers and school authorities at the project site cooperate fully.

During the course of our national study our research team had been on the lookout for a suitable location for the anticipated investigation. After considering several possibilities, we agreed on a cooperative venture between the University of Wisconsin and three independent school districts adjacent to Houston, Texas. The selection was largely based on the responses of the school administration and the teachers to our proposal, the available population of children with educational handicaps, and provision for their education in special classes. Furthermore, the school agreed that we could provide in-service training of the teachers prior to and during the course of the investigation.

We employed a multivariate research design (Rarick, Dobbins, & Broadhead, 1976) that used four treatments or programs of instruction. Two were physical education instructional programs—one individually oriented, the other group oriented. The third program was an art education program, which we used to assess the Hawthorne effect. The fourth was an experimental control, the usual classroom instructional program. The investigation included a total of 481 children in the 49 special education classes in the three school districts—275 children who were educable mentally retarded (EMR) and 206 children who were minimally brain injured (MBI). Thus, there were 25 classes of children who were EMR and 24 classes of children who were MBI, all within the age range of 6 to 13 years. We employed a multivariate analysis of variance and covariance design that permitted the assessment of treatment (program) effects according to disability, age, and sex for each of the measures of motor, cognitive, social, and emotional development.

We used standard tests given at the beginning and end of the experiment to assess changes in the motor, cognitive, social, and emotional development of all subjects. In the motor domain we used dynamometric measures of grip and arm-shoulder strength and an appropriately modified version of the AAHPER Physical Fitness Test. Cognitive development was assessed by the Peabody Picture Vocabulary Test and the Bender Gestalt Test. Sociometric evaluations of peer acceptance and the Cowell Social Behavior Trend Index were used to assess social development. The emotional parameter of development was evaluated by the Cattell Personality Questionnaire and by the emotional indicators from the Bender Gestalt Test.

Classroom teachers taught the experimental programs for some 35 minutes each school day over the 20 weeks of the experiment. Teachers in the three experimental programs received extensive in-service training before the start of the experiment, and regular periodic supervision and consultation were provided by a trained project consultant. The experiences given to the children in the experimental programs were carefully planned and supervised in the two physical education programs by a trained and experienced special physical education teacher, and in the art program by a specialist in art education.

It was evident from the findings that special treatment as afforded by the two physical education programs and the art education program resulted in statistically greater gains in the motor, intellectual, and emotional development of the children who were EMR and brain injured than occurred with the children in the regular instructional program. Of the three experimental programs, the two physical education programs were superior in modifying motor performance. The art program had the greatest impact on improving the emotional development of the younger children, and the three programs had similar roles in modifying the cognitive development of the children. Overall positive changes were more evident in the older than in the younger children, were more frequently manifested by the children who were brain injured than by the children who were EMR, and were marginally more frequently noted in the males than in the females.

Of significance was the effect of the special programs (data pooled across treatments) on measures of motor, intellectual, and emotional development. In other words, special attention, whether relating to the quality of instruction or resulting in undefined motivation of the children, appeared to be a critical factor in altering these aspects of development. Clearly, the positive effect of physical activity programs on measures of intelligence was no greater than that resulting from the art program.

The impact of individualizing instruction was clearly apparent; the changes elicited by the individualized physical education program on the measures of intellectual, social, and emotional development of these children were substantially greater than changes in the children who had group instruction. It is perhaps not surprising that as a group the older children and the children who were MBI profited more than the younger children and the children who were EMR, probably reflecting greater maturity and higher intellectual levels in the former.

The Berkeley Years

My move to the University of California at Berkeley in 1968 in no way reflected any dissatisfaction with the support my work was given at the University of Wisconsin. It was apparent that I could continue my research with equally good support at Berkeley without the rigors of the Wisconsin winters. After much soul searching, I decided to make the change.

By this time much of my research focus had become centered on the motor behavior of exceptional children, primarily children with educational disabilities. Being less than satisfied with the motor tests in use with this population of children and recognizing that our understanding of the organizational structure of their motor abilities was limited, I embarked on a series of studies with these dissatisfactions in mind. Due to space limitations, I will refer here to only two Berkeley investigations, studies that are closely related. In brief, these studies (Rarick, 1980; Rarick et al., 1976) were designed to use factor analytic methods to identify the basic components of motor performance of children and adolescents with mental retardation. Little attention up to this time had been given to ascertaining the extent to which such components, once identified, were common across age, sex, and level of intelligence.

The hypothesis that I proposed to test was that the basic components of motor performance emerging from a factor analysis of a wide range of fine and gross motor tests given to children and adolescents of varying chronological ages and intellectual levels would not differ materially even though the subjects' performance capabilities might vary markedly. The rationale for this hypothesis was based largely on my observations of the motor performances of these individuals, their similarities in anatomical characteristics, and the culture common to them all. Furthermore, a procedure developed by Kaiser, Hunda, and Bianchini (1971) permitted quantitative comparisons of the factor structures of motor performance across age-sex-intellectual levels.

To undertake such a project I needed a sizable sample of boys and girls who were not retarded, in addition to samples of children who were EMR and children who were trainable mentally retarded (TMR) grouped into appropriate age categories of approximately equal number. I also needed the cooperation of school districts within a reasonable geographical area as well as the support of parents. I was able to meet all of these conditions. Trained testers and portable testing facilities posed no problem, because I was able to obtain adequate federal funding for the project.

I was fortunate at the outset to obtain full cooperation of several special and elementary schools in the San Francisco–East Bay region, which provided 145 boys and girls (ages 6-10 years) who were not retarded, 261 boys and girls of two age levels (6-10 years and 10-13 years) who were EMR, and 453 boys and girls of four age levels (6-10 years, 10-14 years, 14-18 years, and 18-21 years) who were TMR. The rationale for using a single age level of children who were not retarded was to provide, for comparative purposes, one group of children with IQ levels approximately the same as those of the older group of children who were EMR.

I formulated a hypothesized factor structure based on previous factor analytic studies of nonretarded adolescents and young adults. See Table 7.1 for a listing of the test items grouped according to hypothesized factors. All testing was done by trained testers at the respective school sites—outdoor testing on school playgrounds, indoor testing in a 10-foot by 55-foot mobile unit.

Table 7.1   Tests Grouped According to Hypothesized Factor Structure of the Motor Domain

I.   Static muscular strength
   1. Grip strength right
   2. Grip strength left
   3. Cybex elbow flexion
   4. Cybex elbow extension
   5. Cybex knee flexion
   6. Cybex knee extension

II.   Explosive muscular strength
   *1. Vertical jump
   2. Standing broad jump
   3. 35-yard dash (35-5)
   4. Bicycle ergometer with resistance (10 sec)
   5. Softball throw (velocity)

III.   Muscular strength-endurance
   1. Sit-ups
   2. Trunk raise for time
   3. Leg raise for time
   4. Bicycle ergometer total (90 sec)

IV.   Gross body coordination
   1. Scramble
   2. Mat crawl
   *3. Tire run
   °4. Zig-zag run
   5. Bicycle ergometer without resistance (10 sec)

V.   Cardiorespiratory endurance
   1. Physical work capacity (170)
   2. 150-yard dash

VI.   Limb-eye coordination
   °1. Pursuit rotor at 10 RPM
   2. Pursuit rotor at 20 RPM
   *3. Pursuit rotor at 40 RPM
   4. Target throw horizontal
   5. Target throw vertical
   °6. Light buttons

VI.   Limb-eye coordination (*cont.*)
   °7. Soccer ball catch
   °8. Round target (ball toss for accuracy)

VII.   Manual dexterity
   1. Minnesota Manipulative Test (preferred and non-preferred)
   2. Purdue Pegboard Test
   *3. 2-plate tapping test
   4. Ring stacking test
   5. Golfball placement test

VIII.   Static balance
   *1. Bass Test
   2. Stabilometer
   3. Stork Test (adapted for TMRs)

IX.   Dynamic balance
   1. Railwalk forward
   2. Railwalk backward
   3. Railwalk sideways

X.   Flexibility
   1. Toe touch
   2. Spinal extension
   3. Spinal rotation
   4. Lateral spinal extension

XI.   Body fat
   1. Triceps skinfold
   2. Subscapular skinfold
   3. Abdominal skinfold

XII.   Body size
   1. Biacromial breadth
   2. Biiliac breadth
   3. Calf girth
   4. Height (cm)
   5. Weight (kg)

Note. Reprinted by permission of the American Alliance for Health, Physical Education, Recreation and Dance, 1900 Association Drive, Reston, VA 22091.

*Used only in EMR study.

°Used only in TMR study.

Upon completion of the data collection, I ran intercorrelations (holding chronological age [CA] constant) among all variables according to chronological age, sex, and disability groups, and I factored the residual intercorrelation matrices using three factor solutions, each solution rotated both orthogonally and obliquely. When I compared the separate solutions, any bias according to solution would be evident. The agreement among solutions based on the pattern of factor loadings was remarkably consistent within each age, sex, and disability group. For a description of the procedures used, see Rarick (1980).

To determine more precisely the extent of agreement among the factor structures of the several groups, I used the previously mentioned procedure (Kaiser et al., 1971), applying the orthogonally rotated incomplete principal components solution. The resulting coefficients are cosines between factor axes, which are identified by the factor loadings (definers). The cosines may be conceptually interpreted as correlation coefficients with a theoretical range of +1.00 to −1.00.

The similarity in the factor structures of the different age-sex groups of children who are not retarded and those who are EMR is evident by the magnitude of the means of the cosines between factor axes, ranging from .70 to .90 (see Table 7.2, page 122). In the case of the TMR groups, the factor structure is similar to that for the nonretarded and EMR groups, four factors being common to both. The means of the cosines between factor axes for the TMR groups, although not as high as with the nonretarded and EMR groups, are nevertheless substantial (see Table 7.3, page 123). These results provide substantial evidence of the similarity of the factor structures of the motor domain of school-age children regardless of age, sex, intelligence, or performance level.

As partial validation of the findings, I employed discriminant analysis to determine the effectiveness of the definers in assigning subjects to their respective age, sex, and disability categories. In each case five definers were sufficient for this purpose. The use of more definers did not materially alter the assignment ratios. In the case of the nonretarded and EMR groups, this procedure correctly assigned 82.5% to 95.5% of the children to their original established groups. With the children who were TMR, the results were not quite as good, the percent correctly assigned ranging from 54% to 93%. In other words, although the factor structures were quite similar across groups, the well-established age, sex, and disability differences in performance were clearly evident when I used the definers of the factor structures to assign subjects to their original groups through discriminant analysis.

These findings, I believe, have considerable significance:

- They indicate that there is a well-defined structure of motor abilities that is characteristic of humans of these age levels regardless of sex, performance, or intellectual level.

Table 7.2   Similarity of the Factor Structures of Different Age-Sex Groups of Normal and EMR Children as Reflected by the Means of the Cosines Derived From the Factor Axes of Each of the Six Comparable Common Factors

Factor	Cosines Mean	SD	Common definers
1. Body fat (dead weight)	0.90	0.05	Weight,* three skinfolds (abdominal, subscapular, triceps),* biiliac breadth°
2. Fine visual-motor coordination	0.79	0.10	Minnesota Manipulative,* ring stacking,* 2-plate tapping°
3. Gross limb-eye coordination	0.72	0.18	Target throw vertical,* target throw horizontal,° softball throw (velocity)°
4. Strength-power	0.77	0.14	Knee flexion and extension,* grip strength left°
5. Leg power-coordination	0.76	0.12	35- and 150-yard dashes,* scramble* (no common definers for older EMR boys)
6. Balance	0.70	0.16	Railwalk forward and backward* (no common definers for older EMR boys and girls)

Note. Reprinted by permission of the American Alliance for Health, Physical Education, Recreation and Dance, 1900 Association Drive, Reston, VA 22091.

*Definer common across all groups.

°Definer common across 5 out of 6 groups.

- They provide a foundation for the development of tests that should faithfully reflect the basic components of motor performance.
- They provide additional insight into the nature of motor abilities for those preparing curricula in physical education.

Concluding Comments

My research over the years has for the most part been field oriented; in some cases I have used the longitudinal approach and in others the cross-sectional method. I learned at an early date that conditions, including the

Table 7.3 Similarity of the Factor Structures of the Seven Age-Sex Groups of TMR Subjects as Reflected by the Means of the Cosines Derived From the Factor Axes of Each of the Seven Comparable Common Factors

Factor	Cosines		Common definers
	Mean	SD	
1. Body fat (dead weight)	0.93	0.04	Weight,* three skinfolds (triceps, subscapular, abdominal),* calf girth,° biiliac breadth°
2. Fine visual-motor coordination	0.76	0.18	Minnesota Manipulative (preferred and nonpreferred hands),* ring stacking (preferred and nonpreferred hands)°
3. Balance	0.64	0.14	Railwalk side and back,* railwalk forward,° stork test (adapted)°
4. Upper limb-eye coordination	0.53	0.30	Target horizontal,* target circle,* target vertical,° ball catch°
5. Arm strength	0.63	0.23	Elbow flexion and extension*
6. Spinal flexibility	0.73	0.13	Lateral spinal extension,* spinal extension°
7. Leg power-coordination	0.43	0.24	Bicycle with and without resistance,* bicycle 90 seconds°

Note. Reprinted by permission of the American Alliance for Health, Physical Education, Recreation and Dance, 1900 Association Drive, Reston, VA 22091.

*Definer common across all groups.

°Definer common across 6 out of 7 groups.

nature of the problem and the population to be studied, dictate which of the two methods is appropriate. Although some of my research has had a theoretical orientation, much has been applied to issues of the times, questions for which testable hypotheses were in some instances appropriate, in others not suitable.

Recently questions have been raised about the orientation of motor development research, namely that it has been primarily product oriented (normative-descriptive) with little emphasis on underlying processes or mechanisms and that the focus has been on *when* (stages of development) rather than on *how* (explanation) (Kelso & Clark, 1982). To infer that this research is essentially devoid of theory (explanation) implies that research in such disciplines as astronomy, anthropology, and archaeology likewise have no theoretical orientation simply because their sources of data do not permit controlled experimentation.

It is true that most of the research in motor development has over the years been normative-descriptive and/or applied in its orientation, but this does not mean it has added little importance to our knowledge base. The search for underlying processes in complex systems, which themselves are undergoing change, is a worthy but difficult task, one that when properly done requires a multidisciplinary approach. Although the need for basic research here is clearly evident, let us not forget the value of applied research. The latter has long been recognized as a vital, creative part of research in universities, and it plays a key role in innovation and as such is an important part of academic research (Clogston, 1987). The answer is not either/or but a healthy balance of the two.

Chapter 8

David A. Sugden

School of Education
University of Leeds
Leeds, England

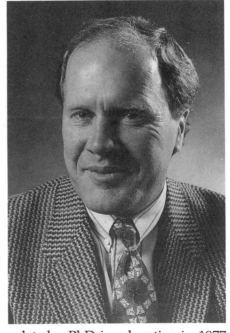

Born in Upton, Yorkshire, England, in 1945, David Sugden received his initial teacher training at Loughborough College of Education, gaining his teaching certificate in 1966. After teaching for 4 years in the English schools system, he moved to the United States, completing BSc and MSc degrees in physical education and kinesiology at UCLA in 1970 and 1972, respectively. Sugden returned to the United Kingdom from 1972 to 1974 to take up a lectureship in the Department of Physical Education at St. Mary's College of Education at Twickenham; then he returned to UCLA from 1974 to 1976 to undertake studies toward a doctorate. He completed a PhD in education in 1977 following supervision by Professors Jack Keogh and F.W. Hewett. During the period of his postgraduate education, Sugden retained his clinical skills in the special education field by teaching at the Los Angeles Exceptional Children's Foundation (1970-72) and at the Martin Luther King Hospital (1974-76). He returned to England in 1976 to a lectureship in psychology and education at St. Mary's College of Education. Sugden moved subsequently to the University of Leeds in 1977 to an appointment in physical education and later, in 1981, to the School of Education at the same institution, where he is today Reader in Motor Development and Impairment.

Dr. Sugden's research work has proceeded largely from within an information-processing framework and has contributed significantly to understanding of the processing capacities and limitations of children who are retarded and those who are not retarded. Using recipient paradigms from the motor learning and control field, Sugden has demonstrated fundamental developmental differences in movement speed and movement control (using Fitts's 1954 reciprocal tapping task) (Sugden, 1980b) and in strategies for the encoding and retrieval of information from visual and motor short-term memory (Sugden, 1980a). He has also used similar paradigms to demonstrate the nature of information-processing, capacity, and strategy deficits in children who are retarded (Sugden, 1978; Sugden & Gray, 1981) and as a basis for developing assessment procedures for motor impairment in this special population (e.g., Sugden & Newall, 1987; Sugden & Wann, 1987). Sugden has also contributed significantly to understanding of the development of proprioception (Sugden, 1986, 1990), although (as is the case with his coauthor and former supervisor Jack Keogh) his two texts on motor development in normal (Keogh & Sugden, 1985) and special populations (Sugden & Keogh, 1990), which summarize much of the thrust of his research career, are likely to be his most enduring and influential works. David Sugden has been a keen rugby player and is a current editorial board member of *Adapted Physical Activity Quarterly*.

David Sugden's chapter provides us with our first autobiographic exposure to the importance of a supervisor/adviser in influencing the research orientation and interests of an experimenter. Sugden notes the influence of Jack Keogh as his mentor, and Sugden's involvement in process-oriented research clearly reflects the direction for motor development research advocated by Keogh in his own chapter (chapter 6). Sugden also provides a good example of someone who primarily uses data-driven research and employs field observations to provide the basis for research hypotheses. Like Rarick in chapter 7, Sugden notes the importance of descriptive research and the mutuality between description and explanation; like a number of other motor development researchers and an increasing number of motor learning and control researchers, Sugden advocates strongly the importance of both naturalistic and longitudinal research. Sugden's concerns regarding the necessary trade-offs between depth and breadth in research training and focus, and his concerns regarding the practical difficulties of keeping abreast with the burgeoning developments in knowledge and technologies in allied fields, touch on very real pragmatic difficulties for experimenters. Note these difficulties carefully; we will examine these in further detail in chapter 14.

AUTOBIOGRAPHY

My research career has been solely concerned with the movement skills of children. My initial training was in physical education, and although this was geared to the child aged 11 years and older, it soon became clear that my interest was with younger children. From general observation of children in movement situations, I have formulated three fundamental questions that have guided my research. First, how can I describe children's movement skill development? Second, how can I account for or explain this development? Third, when movement skill development is obviously impaired, how can I improve it? Unfortunately for me, these areas draw upon such diverse literature and experimental techniques that the common problem of sacrificing depth for breadth becomes a reality.

Observing children in daily movement experiences raises fundamental questions and possible hypotheses. For example, I can try to help one of my children ride a two-wheeled bike at Easter time. I remove the training wheels and spend the next 2 hours holding on to the seat of the bike while she attempts to ride it. We both finish exhausted. The next day, we give the bicycle a miss and start on the garden swing. I spend the session pushing a little and then shouting *pull* at the appropriate times during the swing. Unfortunately, the swinging teaching has as much effect as that for the bicycle. Three months later in the summer, my daughter tells me that she can ride her bike. No practice since Easter, and one-trial success; the same is true of the swinging. What has happened during the 3 months that has facilitated this success? If we had continued practicing at Easter over a period of days, would we have achieved the same result?

Other observations raise as many questions. Take a task like rolling a ball for accuracy, as in playing skittles or trying to be closest to a line or hole. This kind of task requires a minimum level of fitness variables such as strength or speed and does not depend upon body size, yet if we measured children between the ages of 5 and 10 years, we would obtain very clear developmental trends. Older children obviously will have developed some personal resources that aid the performance of this particular task.

In a different vein, if I visit a school for children with moderate learning difficulties and observe a physical education lesson, I will see more children with movement problems than in a classroom of nonretarded children. How many more will depend upon the makeup of the class, but I will see at least twice as many. I will see problems involving skillful movements, and not just those that rely heavily on fitness factors. This higher incidence of problems is not related to any known constitutional problems in the children, because with moderate learning difficulties, known organic problems are not common. So why should there be such a higher incidence of movement problems?

Finally, if I attempt to teach a child a skill with which the child has a movement problem, for example a two-footed jump, how do I set about this? What guidelines do I follow? When the child is successful, what exactly has he or she learned? More important, has the child learned only that skill, or have any general skills been learned?

These observations pose developmental questions, and development involves change over time. Flavell (1970) nicely summarized the kinds of changes that can take place, and although he aimed them at cognitive changes, they provide an equally valid framework for the movement domain. These changes are those of addition, substitution, modification, inclusion, and mediation, and they can be examined in a wide range of experimental paradigms. For example, modification may occur when a child has to adjust his or her walking pattern to different terrain; such modification may require experimental techniques different than inclusion, which involves a child incorporating a movement like finger-thumb opposition into a variety of movements, such as holding a knife or twisting a knob.

In the early 1970s my initiation into research was influenced by a diversity of factors. First, I moved to California where I met Jack Keogh (see chapter 6), who was stressing then that the serious developmental questions were not the height, weight, speed, and strength variables but involved the variables of process. This meeting developed into a professional relationship that has resulted in two books on development and impairment (Keogh & Sugden, 1985; Sugden & Keogh, 1990).

Second, I worked part-time for 4 years at an institution called Exceptional Children's Foundation (ECF), which was a collection of schools for children evidencing all kinds of problems. In my first 2 years I was involved in establishing remedial motor programs, but later I took on a wider brief involving other subject areas. Every day that I worked at ECF I saw a variety of children with movement problems, ranging from children who were nearly immobile to those with movements that were not efficient or graceful.

Finally, at this time I was studying at UCLA and came across a body of literature that sent my thoughts spinning in all directions. On the one hand some of the literature was a little disappointing in that it took motor problems as a secondary presenting condition, or it examined the effect of various motor programs on other abilities such as reading. In the same vein the developmental literature concentrated on growth. However, new approaches were being documented, an example being a text edited by Connolly in 1970 entitled *Mechanisms of Motor Skill Development*. This text became very influential, not because of the new data it presented but because it showed a different way of looking at development. A group of scientists posed questions and raised issues that were novel in this field. This new approach coincided with a surge of interest in the process of skill acquisition in the adult literature, and it was not long before the two were combined.

Thus, with this eclectic mix of selective reading, practical observation, and naive enthusiasm, I embarked upon my first investigation. Working with Jack Keogh and other graduate students at UCLA, I started to investigate the incidence and nature of motor problems in young children. We did this by using three methods: We asked the teachers, we observed the children in their physical education lessons, and we gave the children standardized tests. We obtained some fine data: a range of incidence depending upon the criterion set upon gender differences, and upon children who had more problems in the playground than in the classroom and vice versa. This was exciting research.

However, we then began to examine the results in more detail. We found that the children identified by one method were not necessarily the same as those identified by another. Certainly there was some overlap, but there were also enough differences to cause serious concern. Additionally, when we examined the children 1 year later, we identified different children. Again some children were the same, but some of the original ones had dropped out and new ones picked up (Keogh et al., 1979). These were the real issues of research. What had happened? The testing in all phases had been very carefully controlled, but it is possible that some confounding variables had crept in. More likely, here was evidence of children's known variability, the fact that development begins at different starting points and progresses at different rates and in varying directions. The different forms of assessment were probably examining different functions. These questions involving stability of problems over time and involving multiple assessments still have only been infrequently addressed, and much more work is required (Henderson & Hall, 1982).

At the same time that my interest in the assessment of motor problems was growing, other literature was also guiding my thoughts. I was studying developmental psychology and special education at UCLA and became interested in the cognitive processes of children with mental retardation. Information processing with various models of memory was very popular, and some investigators had used these paradigms with children who were mentally retarded. Memory processes had been found to be poor in these children; in particular, short-term memory was deficient. I had read the various explanations of this deficit from researchers such as Spitz (1966) and Ellis (1963, 1970), but the study that really impressed me was Belmont and Butterfield (1969). Like many older studies, it now appears dated. However, it is an important study, one that was carried out with elegance and rigor. Using number stimuli to remember, and presentation time that could be under the control of subjects, the authors devised a "hesitation time" to indicate whether subjects were mentally rehearsing information that was presented to them. The results were very clear: There was a developmental progression in rehearsal, with young children and the developmentally young (persons who were mentally retarded) having short hesitation times, indicating a lack of rehearsal strategies. In contrast, older children and adults not only hesitated longer, indicating that they were rehearsing the information, but also gave verbal reports that this is what they were in fact doing. This rehearsal was directly related to better performance on the memory task.

Several bodies of knowledge now began to come together for me. First, children who were mentally retarded did not spontaneously use mnemonic strategies on verbal tasks. Second, children who were mentally retarded had poorer motor performance than children who were not retarded. Third, researchers were beginning to perform some interesting memory studies in the motor control area (Laabs, 1973). I used all of these sources to examine visual motor memory and its relationship to age and intelligence (Sugden, 1978). The results were clear in that they mirrored those from the verbal literature. Young and developmentally young children did not spontaneously use mnemonic strategies on a visual motor memory task. Older children did use these strategies, with resultant better memory performances. When older children were prevented from using a mnemonic strategy, their memory performances were no different than those of younger children, confirming Flavell's (1970) proposition that in order for the researcher to obtain developmental differences, the task must allow for developmental strategies.

This type of research was having its final fling in the adult motor skills area at the end of the 1970s, although work with children and mental retardation did continue a little longer (Kelso, Goodman, Stamm, & Hayes, 1979; Reid, 1980). Researchers had moved away from using verbal models to explain motor behavior and were turning their attention to the motor rather than the cognitive side of skilled action. With children there was little experimental evidence in this area, and so I spent a couple of years examining speed-accuracy trade-offs in Fitts's type paradigms. I used both discrete and serial tasks that enabled me to look at such things as programming and feedback time. Results were encouraging in that children's fast movements could be explained in Fitts's terms both for discrete and serial tasks. In addition there were some interesting developmental trends showing older children to be much more capable of programming their movements to run off without recourse to feedback (Sugden, 1980b). We also examined these processes in children who were mentally retarded. We selected 12-year-olds with moderate learning difficulties and with no known physical handicaps or minor congenital anomalies. Yet on the Fitts's task, they performed at levels 3 to 4 years below their chronological ages. They showed similar trends to children who were not retarded, in that the children with mental retardation confirmed Fitts's law, but their times resembled those of younger children (Sugden & Gray, 1981). Thus there was the important finding that in children with moderate learning difficulties with no organic problem, movements were slower to all targets. Why should this be? Possibilities include attention difficulties, capacity problems, and neural problems that have not been detected.

By the beginning of the 1980s, we were finding that children who were mentally retarded were deficient on all information-processing tasks, whether the tasks were cognitive or motor in nature. Some researchers feel this really only takes us back to a different level of description rather than forward to new levels of explanation (Newell, 1985). However, this descriptive gain in itself is important, as is the fact that the division between description and explanation is not as clear-cut as we sometimes suspect. In addition, I find that the answers to my three fundamental questions will only come about through gradual emergence, as I build upon previous work, not through a total abandonment of previous results. Certainly some of the work we did in the early and mid-1970s is dated, yet we have built on this to provide our current directions. One disturbing feature of motor skills research has been an all-or-none approach to investigations. In the 1970s, this was exemplified by the polarized open- and closed-loop stances, whereas more recently many researchers see cognitive processes as an anathema. Some researchers have been brave enough to address questions that have gone out of favor, with valuable debate being the result (Zanone & Hauert, 1987). I can only hope for more in this mold.

For researchers interested in the study of movement development, the summer of 1985 was a landmark. A NATO Advanced Study Institute organized by Mike Wade and John Whiting was held in Maastricht, Holland. This meeting provided the opportunity for those involved in motor development to present papers, exchange ideas, and propose new directions. We were all given topics to present, and mine involved describing the development of proprioception. This was a topic that I had examined when looking at short-term memory, but this presentation gave me the opportunity to take a much closer look. I propose that there are two fundamental ways in which proprioception can be described. The first is proprioceptive perception and is the traditional sensing of movement involving receptors in the joints, muscles, tendons, and ears. The second is the more useful concept of proprioceptive control, which is the totality of the traditional sense plus vision acting proprioceptively, and together the total system is linked to action. Developmentally, this has important implications, because there is evidence that very early in life, infants use the equivalences between visual and proprioceptive information as a basis for organizing their responses (Meltzoff & Moore, 1985). This information is not exclusively visual or proprioceptive, and although it is nonmodality specific, the description of an event is multisensory in nature and is ripe for development both in the form of integration and differentiation.

During the early years of childhood, children modify their earlier achievements, leading to a large repertoire of movement skills. There are developmental milestones beyond infancy, but more often the child varies the movement, in different ways, often in novel situations. Children acquire finer control of their own movements and learn how to control them in relation to moving others or objects. It is not unreasonable to suggest that the development of proprioception is a contributing factor to these changes in skill development; however, one has to ask what form this contribution takes. For example, will an increase in proprioceptive ability be accompanied by a similar rise in skill level? Taking this a little further, one can ask whether improving the proprioceptive level of a child with known movement problems will aid the child's skill level. I recently investigated the first part of this question by examining proprioceptive ability in children with and without known motor problems. I used a published proprioceptive test (Laszlo & Bairstow, 1985) and a test of motor impairment (Stott, Moyes, & Henderson, 1984) and examined a group of children with moderate learning difficulties. My aim was to discover the relationship between the two tests. Unfortunately this relationship was not very strong. Some children performed poorly on the functional test and yet were satisfactory for the group on the test of proprioception. Some were very poor on the proprioceptive test and yet passed the functional test. Obviously others were poor on both tests, but overall the results were not clear (Sugden & Wann, 1987). I believe that this says a lot more about the measure we used than about the relationship of proprioception to skill performance. The test of proprioception involved only a passive discrimination task in a nonvision condition, plus a cross-modal task, again passively presented. Thus, we were testing proprioceptive perception rather than any multimodal description of an event. The assessment only tapped a small part of what we know is proprioceptive control. The functional test, on the other hand, not only tapped a wider range of proprioceptive skills but also showed that these skills may only make up a small part of the total variance of the task.

What are the future directions of developmental research? Certainly the three fundamental questions I asked at the beginning still need to be addressed. Our approaches, however, are changing, with more naturalistic settings being used. A movement does not take place in isolation: It is the result of the transaction between the personal resources of the mover, the setting in which the movement takes place, and the task to be performed. Movement skills are context determined and context specific. Our technology has improved so much in the last 10 years that we can now use various recording techniques that will enable us to use these naturalistic settings.

These naturalistic settings are particularly important for developmental investigations that examine the change process. We can investigate this change by using longitudinal methods and following a group of children over a period of years. However, most of us are not afforded that kind of luxury, and we have to fall back on the cross-sectional study. This is unfortunate, because by using different children at different ages, we are making considerable inferences about development. In the movement skill area we have few longitudinal studies, most of which are concerned with anthropometric variables. Certainly a major step forward would be for us to obtain longitudinal data on how children learn movement skills as opposed to the more simplistic performance studies that have prevailed. We are now really beginning to ask developmental questions concerning the change process rather than simply using adult paradigms with children, or employing children as subjects because they may throw light on general skill processes.

Chapter 9

Jerry R. Thomas

Department of Exercise Science and Physical Education
Arizona State University
Tempe, Arizona, U.S.A.

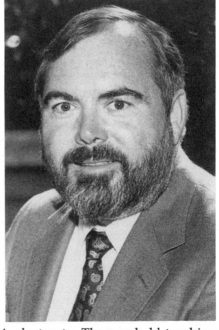

J erry Thomas was born in 1941 and completed his undergraduate degree, a BA in physical education, at Furman University in 1963. This was followed in 1964 by an MA from the University of Alabama, and in 1970 by an EdD with a major in physical education and minors in research and statistics and child development from the same institution. His doctoral dissertation involved a study of instructional grouping, motor ability, and interpersonal relationships of 6th-grade boys, and he completed his graduate education while holding a variety of physical education positions in the public schools and in state and junior college systems. After completing his doctorate, Thomas held teaching and research positions at Georgia Southern College (1970-73), Florida State University (1973-77), and Louisiana State University (1977-88) before moving to his current position as professor and chair of the Department of Exercise Science and Physical Education at Arizona State University. Jerry Thomas played football at college and has since turned his sporting skills to golf and softball.

Dr. Thomas's contributions to the current knowledge base in the motor development field and to the general development of the physical education/ kinesiology discipline and profession have been many and varied. His initial work involved examining the relationship between perceptual-motor and academic performance in children (e.g., J.R. Thomas & Chissom, 1972, 1974a, 1974b). This topic, as Jack Keogh noted in chapter 6, was of practical importance to educators because putative links between motor and perceptual development and between perception and cognition were being used, at the time, as the rationale for a range of remediation programs.

Thomas's most enduring contributions to knowledge (made following the studies on motor-intellectual relationships) have involved testing the applicability of a range of mainstream cognitive theories of development within the motor context. Thomas has conducted extensive empirical tests on the explanatory power of neo-Piagetian theories (e.g., Gerson & Thomas, 1977; J.R. Thomas & Bender, 1977); of cognitive models of strategy development, especially those based on encoding strategies for motor short-term memory (e.g., Gallagher & Thomas, 1980, 1984, 1986; J.R. Thomas, 1980; J.R. Thomas, Thomas, Lee, Testerman, & Ashy, 1983); and of knowledge-based approaches to expertise (e.g., French & Thomas, 1987; McPherson & Thomas, 1989; J.R. Thomas, French, & Humphries, 1986). His original contribution to knowledge has also extended to research work on the development of gender differences in motor performance (e.g., J.R. Thomas & French, 1985; J.R. Thomas & Nelson, 1991), to methodological issues related to meaningfulness of findings (J.R. Thomas, Salazar, & Landers, 1991) and appropriate handling of error score analysis (J.R. Thomas, 1977a), and to the potential role of meta-analysis in studies of human action (J.R. Thomas & French, 1986).

In addition to his contributions to knowledge in the motor development field, he has also written extensively on the discipline and its direction (e.g., J.R. Thomas, 1987a, 1990, 1991); his general texts on research methods (J.R. Thomas & Nelson, 1985, 1990) and physical education for children (e.g., J.R. Thomas, Lee, & Thomas, 1988a, 1988b), as well as an edited volume on motor development (J.R. Thomas, 1984), have been influential at the broadest level. Jerry Thomas, like many of the expert experimenters included in this book, has also made substantial contributions to the profession, most notably as editor of the *Research Quarterly for Exercise and Sport* (1983-89) and as president of NASPSPA (1990-91). In recognition of his contributions to the profession and to original knowledge, Dr. Thomas has been honored with fellowship of the American Academy of Physical Education and elected president, 1992-93, given the Honor Award (1990), and honored as alliance scholar of the American Alliance for Health, Physical Education, Recreation and Dance (in 1989-90).

Jerry Thomas, in this chapter, gives us a first-person perspective on the events and cognitions that have marked his career in experimentation and that have taken him through a range of theoretical and paradigmatic positions to his current focus on naturalistic research on expertise. The chapter not only provides a rationale for the importance of studying real-world phenomena (see also J.R. Thomas, 1989) but also chronicles the prevalence of problem-driven research even among expert experimenters. Thomas notes that although there has been some transition in his orientation from problem-driven to theory-driven research as his career has developed, the theoretical context, in practice, has often been applied in a post hoc fashion. This chapter also provides us (in Thomas's studies of gender differences) with an excellent example of method-driven experimentation, research for which the stimulus for experimentation was the availability of a new method (meta-analysis) rather than the availability of theory or unexplained data.

AUTOBIOGRAPHY

"Some of the most important discoveries have been made without any plan of research . . . there are researchers who do not work on a verbal plane, who cannot put into words what they are doing."

RICHTER, 1953, pp. 91-92

This statement, made almost 40 years ago by Richter, suggests that experts may not always know how they do the things that make them expert. That observation has support in more current studies of the development of expertise (e.g., Adelson, 1984). In recent years my interest has focused on how the development of expertise occurs in children's skill performance. Thus, I think it is most appropriate to point out at the beginning of a chapter in which I am to share my "expertise" as a movement scientist that I may not, in fact, know how I do the things that have allowed me (and I hope continue to allow me) to develop and investigate problems that have scientific merit to other scholars. If you were to ask my graduate students how to formalize my scientific method, they might give (and often have given) the following account:

1. Select good graduate students.
2. Have them read and study the literature.
3. Pick their minds for good ideas.
4. Jointly develop experiments to test the ideas.
5. Instruct them to collect the data.
6. Place my name on the papers as the first author.
7. Make the students find dissertation topics on top of everything else.

However, I choose not to give validity to such an unconscionable account, first formulated by my wife but subsequently espoused by others.

For you to understand how I do what I do, some background is important. My graduate work, although with fine, professional individuals, was at an institution (University of Alabama) not noted for scholarship in human movement science or for producing researchers. However, I had some educational experiences that contributed to my interest in scholarship. First, I was exposed to the value of research as an undergraduate at Furman University by Ruth Reid and W.L. Carr. Second, in my doctoral work at the University of Alabama, I acquired minors in both child development and educational statistics. Thus, although my knowledge base about human movement was somewhat limited—to be truthful, at that time everyone's was—I had a focus on developmental processes and the skills needed in experimental design and statistical analysis. Further, I had considerable interests in practical aspects of children's skill acquisition, which resulted from several years as an elementary physical education teacher. To summarize, I had a focus (children's skill acquisition), a perspective (developmental), and a set of skills (experimental design and statistics). One might categorize me at that point as a rather good technician in search of a question. However, finding a question was no easy task, and it required me to stumble around trying to develop a sound knowledge base about how children acquire skill. In fact, if I have a single point to make from this chapter, it is that developing knowledge about how children acquire skill is the key to formulating meaningful and valuable research questions about motor development. Such questions do not grow out of methodology or statistics; they come from knowing everything possible about how children learn and from having the intense drive to know more and understand it better.

Early Work

Early in my career I devoted a considerable period of time to acquire a sound knowledge base about how children acquire movement skill. The graduate program I went through did not emphasize the need for a focused and theoretical basis in a specialized area. Thus, I began my work in what was a dead-end area of investigation—the relation between perceptual-motor and academic function in children (J.R. Thomas & Thomas, 1986). I do not mean to suggest that the study of cognition in motor skill acquisition is not an important issue; here I am specifically referring to attempts to show that academic performance is related to and can be improved by perceptual-motor function (e.g., Cratty, 1972; Frostig & Horne, 1964; Kephart, 1960).

Obviously however, I failed to recognize that this was not a particularly good line of research to develop. Working closely with a colleague, Brad

Chissom, we followed the approved model of scientific inquiry—describe, predict, and explain. Initial studies (Chissom, Thomas, & Collins, 1974; J.R. Thomas & Chissom, 1972; J.R. Thomas, Chissom, & Biasiotto, 1972) explored and described the relation between certain types of perceptual-motor skills and academic performance. The following example may shed some light on how sophisticated our problem-solving techniques were. Brad and I had done considerable pilot work in selecting perceptual-motor tasks and exploring how they related to academic performance. We had used many of the traditional tasks such as balance, eye-hand coordination, and so forth. But we still lacked a task we considered to have all the important characteristics necessary to successfully predict academic performance. One evening while we were sitting in Brad's den discussing the problem, his 4-year-old son Russ was playing with a Tupperware toy called the Shape-O-Ball. This toy requires that shapes of different sizes be placed into corresponding holes in the surface of the ball. As I watched Russ playing with this toy, I noted to Brad that the toy required all the characteristics in which we were interested: fine eye-hand coordination, shape recognition, and perceptual-motor matching. Further, we could develop a test by recording the amount of time required for a child to place all the pieces in the correct holes. In the studies previously cited, the Shape-O-Ball test was the single best predictor of academic readiness and performance in young children. As phrased by our "friends," the Thomas-Chissom cookie cutter (so named because the pieces from the Shape-O-Ball test were sometimes used to cut different shaped cookies) was off to the races (translated in academic terms, multiple studies and publications). So much for logical scientific reasoning.

After showing that our perceptual-motor variables were related to academic performance and readiness, we were ready to see if we could predict future performance and manipulate the perceptual-motor characteristics to influence academic performance and readiness. To abruptly end a line of inquiry, the answer was *no*. Our perceptual-motor measures did not predict future academic performance 1 year later (J.R. Thomas & Chissom, 1974a), nor did changing perceptual-motor characteristics by training result in improved academic readiness and performance (J.R. Thomas, Chissom, Stewart, & Shelley, 1975). However, providing additional evidence that this approach was not a useful one was worthwhile, because the topic was of substantial interest to clinicians and teachers. In fact, substantial amounts of money were being invested in perceptual-motor training programs by schools and individuals. Even more recently the topic has attracted enough interest to warrant a chapter (J.R. Thomas & Thomas, 1986) debunking this approach. Books are still being published that propose perceptual-motor training as a means of increasing academic performance (see our book review, J.R. Thomas & Thomas, 1987).

Although these studies represented somewhat of a dead end as a research line, benefits did occur from the work:

1. Brad and I were promoted and tenured from the work.
2. We both got better jobs, Brad at Texas A&M and me at Florida State.
3. I found out a lot about the practical dos and don'ts of experiments with children.
4. I got a chance to use some of the multivariate techniques I had learned on real data.
5. Brad gave me a bronzed Shape-O-Ball engraved with our publication citations.
6. I decided that the development of skilled movement should have value for its own sake and did not need to be justified by the possibility that it might enhance academic performance.

From a scholarly and philosophical perspective, Item 6 was most important; from a practical perspective, Items 1 and 2 were most important.

Memory Development and Motor Performance

At this point several events occurred that influenced my research direction. It was obvious to me that following the research line relating perceptual-motor skill and academic function was pointless. So I began to think about how my interest in skilled performance and my graduate preparation in child development might fit together. At the same time I moved to a new position at Florida State University. This move provided a valuable opportunity for me to work with Bob Singer, who has contributed chapter 4 to this book. Bob's very productive career in motor learning and several of his graduate students influenced me toward a developmental learning model. However, my child development background still directed me toward a stage view of children's learning and performance.

At that point Pascual-Leone's adaptation of Piagetian stage theory to a learning perspective was beginning to draw attention (Pascual-Leone & Smith, 1969). It seemed to me that this model offered considerable promise as a means of explaining children's learning and memory for movements. Working with several graduate students at Florida State, I began a series of investigations using this neo-Piagetian model. In very simple terms, Pascual-Leone's approach suggested that children move from one Piagetian stage to the next as a result of increased capacity in working memory (called *mental space*, or *M-space*). For example, according to Pascual-Leone, a child at the late preoperational stage has the memory capacity of an executive scheme (overall plan) plus two schemes (called figurative or operative), whereas a child at the early concrete stage has the capacity of an executive plus three schemes. Because each scheme represents a unit of information, schemes range from 1 to 7 (seven being Miller's magic number, but for another perspective on Miller, see J.R.

Thomas, 1987b), according to Pascual-Leone's version of Piagetian stages (and substages). Pascual-Leone explained within-stage variability (individual differences) by a test that identified children as high and low M-processors according to their tendencies to use all of their available M-space. The third aspect of his theory was a logical analysis that allowed a task (the problem the child was trying to solve) to be divided into figurative and operative schemes. The model was very attractive because it offered an explanation of the three aspects of development: capacity changes across stages (ages), individual differences within stages, and matching ability with task difficulty.

In a series of published studies (Gerson & Thomas, 1977, 1978; J.R. Thomas & Bender, 1977) and dissertations (Bender, 1976; Mitchell, 1977), we tested several aspects of Pascual-Leone's model with regard to memory for and learning of movement. These studies showed considerable promise when movement tasks were discrete so that we could perform the appropriate task analysis. However, tasks involving more continuous movements were extremely difficult to analyze in the cognitive schemes that were controlling them, particularly as skill increased across trials. Pascual-Leone's theory allowed for separate units to be put together through practice (called accommodation, assimilation, and reciprocal assimilation), thus allowing practice to reduce task demands. The point at which this occurred turned out to be difficult to determine in continuous tasks, especially across acquisition trials.

About the same time, with other graduate students, I began pursuing another approach to explaining changes in children's skill acquisition across age. In several papers (J.R. Thomas, Mitchell, & Solmon, 1979; J.R. Thomas & Moon, 1976; J.R. Thomas, Pierce, & Ridsdale, 1977; J.R. Thomas & Stratton, 1977), two dissertations (Moon, 1975; Stratton, 1977), and one thesis (Pierce, 1977), colleagues and I started work on a developmental view of children's information processing as a means to explain age-related changes in memory for and learning of movement (for a summary, see J.R. Thomas, 1980). This approach was more useful as a model. We gained some preliminary information suggesting that age differences in motor performance were related to use of strategy and rehearsal rather than to capacity changes (as suggested by neo-Piagetian models). This approach was robust across different types of motor tasks (e.g., continuous rhythmic arm movement, balance, and linear positioning).

Following models and approaches developed by Chi (1976) and Ornstein (1978), Jere Gallagher (a graduate student) and I began a series of studies (Gallagher, 1980; Gallagher & Thomas, 1980, 1984, 1986) focused on specific working memory processes that could be manipulated to influence the motor performance of younger and older children. Shortly, Kathi Winther (later to become my wife, K.T. Thomas) joined our research efforts in this area (K.T. Thomas, 1981; J.R. Thomas et al., 1983; Winther & Thomas, 1981). In a series of studies we looked at age differences in rehearsal, organization, and labeling and at how these memory processes could be manipulated to enhance younger children's performance. The findings were robust across ballistic movements, linear positioning in one and two dimensions, and remembering the distance jogged. Further, we were able to demonstrate that the source of the differences was due, at least in part, to working memory attributes as opposed to motor output variability (K.T. Thomas & Thomas, 1988); children may be more variable in motor output, but that did not account for all the differences in performance. In addition, one of my PhD students (Dayan, 1986; Dayan & Thomas, in press) was able to demonstrate that children do not automatically encode the developmental use of spatial information in recalling movement but require considerable effort to remember spatial location (as opposed to the view of Hasher & Zacks, 1979). This finding seems particularly important when we consider the parameters of the movement plan to be learned.

Thus, we were able to demonstrate that a major source of the differences in motor performance between younger and older children and adults is due to differential use of general processes in working memory such as rehearsal, labeling, and organization. Although young children do not necessarily use these processes to aid in memory and performance of movement, they can use them to enhance performance when cued to do so. These findings, if applicable to real teaching and learning situations, suggest actions teachers may take to enhance the ability of younger children to acquire skill. Further, the results suggest that teachers do not have to wait for children to reach specific stages in order to teach certain skills and strategies. Nearly any school-age child can learn the fundamental movements, games, and sports of childhood if the teacher structures the environmental circumstances appropriately and provides good cues and feedback (for a review, see J.R. Thomas & Gallagher, 1986).

However, these studies all had at least two shortcomings (considerably more, some people may argue, but they are all men and women of ill repute). The studies used novel (even trivial) movements under carefully controlled conditions, and the studies did not generalize to more real-world sport settings (J.R. Thomas et al., 1986). Much laboratory research failed to generalize, but the use of novel movements posed a unique problem. By using novel movements we were studying skill acquisition only during the early stages of learning, yet children acquire sport skills over thousands of trials spread across years of practice. Further, ample evidence can be observed that skilled children (experts) perform better than unskilled adults (novices), especially in sports and games for which strength and size are less important factors. Thus, clearly real-world performances do not change in orderly ways across childhood and adolescence. Shifting to a paradigm that involves studying children in real-world sport settings to understand the development of expertise required a major shift in my thoughts, approach, designs, and measurement tools.

Developing Expertise in Sport

I had been interested in youth sport on an applied level for some time; my interest ranged from watching and coaching my son to editing the first manual (Thomas, 1977b) in the United States for youth sport coaches that was derived from the motor development knowledge base. The shift in my focus to development of expertise in sport provided the perfect opportunity for me to combine a very real applied interest with my ongoing research efforts. My first attempt was to outline the general questions of interest (J.R. Thomas et al., 1986, p. 268).

• *How do experts and novices differ in sport knowledge base, specific sport skills, and actual game performance?* Clearly the purpose of this question is to establish descriptive data about specific group differences.

• *What is the relation between sport knowledge, specific sport skills, and game performance?* This question establishes, within specific sports, the variables that are related and thus the ones that should be evaluated as explanations for change.

• *How does one become more competent in game performance?* Although this may not be the basis for true experimental research, it does suggest what should be studied in quasi-designs to evaluate change.

• *What are some of the moderating variables that influence the first, second and third questions?* The performer's age? Amount of past experience? Influence of parents and peers? Characteristics of the teacher or coach?

Although these questions did not exhaust the topic, they established a direction for me to follow in cooperative research efforts with three of my graduate students (French, 1985; Humphries, 1986; McPherson, 1987).

But first we had to develop a new set of technical skills. We wanted to be able to assess performances of children in real-world sport settings. Rather than reinvent the wheel, we adapted some current practices of our colleagues in pedagogy—observing (sometimes live and sometimes by videotape) and coding the performances of interest. However, this requires extensive knowledge of the specific sport. It was necessary to identify important skills and decisions made within the game context. Then we had to develop a system for coding the behaviors of interest that was valid and reliable. Because our interest also included the assessment of the sport knowledge base (declarative: facts, and procedural: how to do something), of sport skills, and of demographic data about children, coaches, and parents, it was necessary for us to find or develop knowledge tests, skill tests, and interview techniques.

French (1985; basketball), Humphries (1986; baseball), and McPherson (1987; tennis) each had to identify, develop, or learn the following:

- An appropriate knowledge test (declarative knowledge) for the sport that was valid and reliable
- Interview techniques about the sport setting, which were used to assess procedural knowledge about how skills are used during performance
- Questionnaires for children, parents, and coaches, which were used to determine necessary demographic data
- Valid and reliable sport skills tests
- Appropriate videotaping skills
- A coding system for the characteristics of interest during game performance that was valid and reliable

Findings from these studies were quite interesting. Portions of French's (1985) dissertation are now published (French & Thomas, 1987) and serve as an example. Experts and novices were different on knowledge, skills, game performance, and procedural situation interviews. Knowledge was most highly related to decision making during game performance, whereas skill tests were most highly related to execution during the game. Over the course of a basketball season, game performance of individuals improved. However, the change was in knowledge and it remained related to decisions at the end of the season. Motor skills did not change and were not related to execution at the end of the season.

McPherson (1987; dissertation is also published, McPherson & Thomas, 1989) reported similar results but also looked at the structure of knowledge in tennis experts and novices. Although experts and novices differed somewhat on declarative knowledge, the most pronounced differences were in procedural knowledge. Experts had more procedures, and these were linked together to form "super" procedures. In addition this study provides the first evidence concerning what we have called an "if-then-do" procedure. In the cognitive area the "then-do" parts of a procedure are nearly perfectly correlated because the "do" part is usually rather simple. However, in sport skills, there may be a considerable difference between a performer's intentions and what he or she actually does. McPherson provided the first indications of how this develops in expert children tennis players. She was able to obtain this information by holding brief interviews between points in tennis matches (while the players were retrieving the tennis balls). Of course this technique could not be used in more continuous sports like soccer and basketball. We have recently summarized this and other related work (J.R. Thomas, French, Thomas, & Gallagher, 1988).

Finding out what experts do is no easy task. First, with well-learned (automated) procedural knowledge and skill, experts often cannot tell you what they do. However, by studying expertise as it develops in children we may be able to observe the process of proceduralization, that is, procedures and super procedures being formed. This seems to be particularly informative when we look at experts who can do what they intend at times but not at other times. Of course in this sense, expertise is always a relative term—a 10-year-old expert may not be as expert as a 13-year-old expert. Innovative techniques like those used by McPherson (1987) let us see developing expertise. By understanding how skillful performance is developed, we can learn more effective ways to help novices become more skilled. If we can combine understanding these processes with increased understanding of expertise in teachers and coaches (e.g., Berliner, 1986), helping children become more skillful performers may become a reality.

Development of Gender Differences in Motor Performance

You might judge at this point that I was methodologically driven in my initial work but that in recent years I have developed a sound theoretical base and have been more theory driven. That is a correct conclusion, for the most part, but not completely. I have always had an interest in new approaches and techniques. As a result of teaching an advanced research methods course to PhD students, I became interested in meta-analysis. Glass's (1977) initial paper offered a straightforward technique (although quite innovative and well thought out). This work aroused substantial interest in the technique, and a subsequent book was published by Glass, McGaw, and Smith (1981). After reading this material and teaching it in research methods, I wanted to try it out; again I had a methodology in search of a question. However, this time I knew what question I wanted to answer and who I needed to help answer it. Karen French was one of my graduate students and was skilled in the quantitative area. We had discussed the development of gender differences in motor performance and whether there might be some way to tease out the underlying causes. Thus, I convinced Karen to learn with me the meta-analysis techniques and apply them to the gender differences question. Of course, if either Karen or I had realized what was going to be involved, we might have given up the idea.

We spent a summer reading and learning Glass's techniques and then began to locate the literature (of course that part was Karen's job because she was the graduate student and I was the professor). We spent about 6 months locating, reading, coding, and analyzing the literature. In fact we had already made one presentation on the results (Thomas & French, 1984) when we encountered Larry Hedges's work on meta-analysis. As we began to read it (for complete presentation, see Hedges & Olkin, 1985), we started to feel that Glass's original techniques were not the most appropriate to handle our data. Karen and I struggled with Hedges's work for about 4 months before finally recognizing that there were parts we couldn't handle. Fortunately, Larry Hedges was doing a 1-day symposium on meta-analysis before the American Educational Research Association meeting in New Orleans (1984). After a phone call to him, Karen went to the symposium, and Larry spent over an hour after the meeting helping her with our problem. Things went much better after that, and the paper we developed was published in *Psychological Bulletin* (J.R. Thomas & French, 1985) and has been my most frequently requested paper. The meta-analysis technique allowed us to infer that nearly all of the gender differences in motor performance observed prior to puberty were environmentally induced but that throwing might be an exception because the differences between boys and girls were so great and appeared so early. A subsequent follow-up study (Nelson, Thomas, Nelson, & Abraham, 1986) substantiated our speculation in that the amount of arm muscle, joint robustness, and shoulder/hip ratio were biological factors that in part accounted for gender differences in throwing at 5 years of age (for a more general review, see J.R. Thomas & Thomas, 1988). This finding was substantiated in a longitudinal follow-up (Nelson, Thomas, & Nelson, 1991). In addition, we (J.R. Thomas & Marzke, 1992) have recently provided an argument for a connection between gender differences in throwing and human evolution. Also, all of the time we spent learning Hedges's techniques for meta-analysis was rewarded in and of itself, as there was substantial interest in our tutorial on the topic (J.R. Thomas & French, 1986) as well as on the use of effect size as an estimate of meaningfulness (J.R. Thomas, Salazar, & Landers, 1991).

Conclusions (Are There Any?)

What can be concluded from this rambling discourse through the research life of Jerry Thomas? I hope one thing is obvious: I truly want to understand how children learn skill and what I can do to make the process easier and more fun. After some wandering around early in my career due to lack of focus in my doctoral work, I spent several years attempting to fathom the underlying cognitive processes that can aid children in learning motor skills. I currently believe that although the information I obtained was useful and valid, I can learn more by studying the skills of interest as they are found in the real world of sport and movement. That does not mean I believe all laboratory research lacks value, just that I think better answers can be found using real-world skills and settings.

Another conclusion (at least for me) is that becoming a productive scholar requires good and dedicated graduate students. You might note the number of joint publications I have with my graduate students. This is because I involve them in my scholarly activities from the beginning. I believe that using a mentor model is the only successful way of preparing quality scholars.

This means daily interactions with graduate students. It also means I can only handle one or two graduate students at a time. The publications and presentations that arise from this model benefit me and the graduate students. The model allows me to investigate and direct investigations into areas that I think have promise and are interesting (at least to me). Graduate students learn the day-to-day skills of planning research, collecting and analyzing data, solving problems, and writing and presenting papers. Graduate students also end up with publications and presentations that aid them in obtaining a position after their graduate work is complete.

However, a mentor model does have one problem. Initially, the professor supplies the ideas and directions for research. But I find I must gradually wean graduate students so that they are generating ideas and I am serving as a colleague and adviser. By the time graduate students are ready to pursue dissertations, they should be independent scholars who have their own lines of research that they can follow when I am no longer available every day. Unless I am careful, or the graduate student is aggressive, it is easy for me to keep on supplying ideas and for the graduate student to continue accepting them.

Finally, it should be obvious that my research is not a neat, theoretically driven model. I attempt to maintain a theoretical basis because I believe a research line has a greater chance of making a long-term contribution if driven by theory. However, sometimes what I do is methodologically derived. I don't know whether the meta-analysis on the development of gender differences in motor performance (J.R. Thomas & French, 1985) was my best paper (it is certainly the most requested) but clearly it developed out of my interest and fascination with the methodology of meta-analysis. In addition, sometimes I conduct a study just because I want to know about something I have observed about children's motor behavior. I will typically put the study within some type of theoretical framework, but that may not be what prompted the work. Further, I find my interest in more recent years (some say because I am getting older) moving toward more generic concerns. For example, after many years of teaching research methods, I felt the need to write a book (J.R. Thomas & Nelson, 1985, 1990) presenting the way I approach this topic for beginning masters students. In addition I have recently completed two books in which colleagues and I attempt to develop a complete package for elementary physical education. This involved using motor development knowledge as the basis for program planning in elementary physical education (J.R. Thomas, Lee, & Thomas, 1988a) and then developing a complete set of lesson plans from this conceptual base (J.R. Thomas, Lee, & Thomas, 1988b). This interest could be just the need to interpret for others what I have spent 15 to 20 years doing, but I also seem to be increasingly concerned about the direction the discipline of human movement and profession of physical education are taking (J.R. Thomas, 1985, 1987a, 1990, 1991). Or maybe Dick Schmidt (1975) was right; inconsistency (variability of practice) is a virtue.

Part IV

Autobiographies in Sport and Exercise Psychology

Although sport and exercise psychology can be satisfactorily defined as that field of study in which the theories and methods of psychology are applied to understanding the behaviors and cognitions of individuals and groups in sport and exercise situations, the clear delimitation of the scope of the field is made difficult by the parent discipline's own difficulties in defining its subject matter (Kendler, 1981; Koch, 1969) and the different connotations of the term *sport psychology* within Europe and North America (Salmela, 1981, 1984). The European view of sport psychology is very broad; according to this view the field encompasses any sport-related research involving the methods and theories of psychology. The European focus is very applied, conceptually tidy, and closely linked to the parent discipline, but its subject matter overlaps heavily with the motor learning and control and motor development fields. The North American view, in contrast, attempts to distinguish sport and exercise psychology from the other human action fields. This orientation has resulted in a field of study that consists of a somewhat odd assortment of historically privileged topics. Information on topics that focus on the psychology of the individual athlete (especially personality, motivation and arousal, anxiety, and attention) and topics that examine sport within the context of social interaction (e.g., social facilitation, leadership and group cohesion, aggression, and sport socialization) form the major knowledge base within the sport psychology field in North America, although we have seen a recent broadening of focus to include issues related to exercise, especially exercise adherence and the psychological effects of exercise.

The modern field of sport and exercise psychology has importance at both the theoretical and practical levels. At the theoretical level, sport psychology serves as an important testing ground for the applicability and generalizability of both mainstream and intrinsically developed psychological theory. At the practical level, problems related to such issues as sport participation, participant and crowd violence, exercise adherence, group cohesion, and performance enhancement remain of persistent interest to sport and exercise practitioners.

The early history of European sport psychology is not well documented, but in North America starting in the 1800s, the Rev. William Augustus Stearn and others wrote about the role of sport and physical activity in promoting mental health and moral development (e.g., see Leonard & Afflect, 1947). The first experimental work in sport psychology is generally considered to be Norman Triplett's work on social facilitation; in this work the author compared the performance of trained cyclists racing against each other and racing against the clock (Triplett, 1898). This was followed by experimental work by W.G. Anderson (1899) on the effectiveness of mental training for skill acquisition and strength development. Systematic programs of sport psychology research followed; facilities in Carl Diem's laboratory in Berlin and in A.C. Puni's laboratory in Leningrad were apparently established by 1920 (Wiggins, 1984). The forebear of American sport psychology was Coleman Griffith (Kroll & Lewis, 1970). Griffith established laboratory facilities for sport psychology research at the University of Illinois in 1925, and the formal course on sport psychology he taught at that institution beginning in 1923 formed the basis for the first English language texts on sport psychology, *Psychology of Coaching* in 1926 and *Psychology and Athletics* in 1928. Griffith's laboratory, which was equipped much like a motor learning and control laboratory of the 1970s (with apparatus for measuring reaction time and kinesthesis), was highly productive until it was closed in 1932 for financial reasons (Kroll & Lewis, 1970).

Although some research on the relationship between physical and mental performance continued in the late 1920s and into the 1930s (e.g., Cozens, 1927; McCloy, 1930; O'Neal, 1936), sport psychology essentially remained dormant in North America until its reemergence after World War II as an offshoot of motor learning and control (Ryan, 1981). Graduates of the motor learning and control programs of Franklin Henry (at Berkeley), John Lawther (at Pennsylvania State University), and Arthur Slater-Hammel (at University of Indiana), in particular, were instrumental in establishing sport psychology as a field of study in its own right. Sport psychology research in the postwar era, not surprisingly, shared the emphasis on controlled laboratory experimentation and measurement precision that preoccupied motor learning and control researchers of the time. The work on stress and motor performance by graduates from Henry's laboratory (e.g., Carron, 1968; Ryan, 1961) and by Celeste Ulrich (e.g., Ulrich, 1957) was typical of the period, although Warren Johnson's works on aggression and personality were equally influential (e.g., Johnson, 1949; Johnson & Hutton, 1955). Due to a growing research base, texts devoted to sport psychology reappeared (e.g., Cratty, 1964; Lawther, 1951) and professional societies were formed, some in conjunction with the other fields of human action research. The International Society of Sport Psychology was formed in 1965, NASPSPA in 1967, and the Canadian Society for Psychomotor Learning and Sport Psychology in 1969 (Loy, 1974; Wiggins, 1984).

The research work of 1950 to 1965 was primarily empirical in nature and was dominated by a glut of largely atheoretical and inconclusive research on sport personality (see Carron, 1980, and Rushall, 1975b, for reviews). In contrast, and largely in response to the inadequacies of the personality research of the preceding era, sport psychology researchers from the mid-1960s through the late 1970s not only diversified their research interests but also became more concerned with theory testing (Landers, 1983). Theories from mainstream social and experimental psychology were liberally tested in the sport context, where issues as diverse as social facilitation and reinforcement, the arousal-performance relationship, modeling, achievement motivation, and attributon theory attracted research attention. Productive programs of research developed in a number of institutions, with the contributions of Dan Landers and Rainer Martens to the general research profile of the field being particularly influential (Ryan, 1981).

Contemporary sport and exercise psychology research maintains an emphasis on a number of the privileged topics of the 1960s and 1970s, albeit with a more situation-specific approach to measurement (Feltz, 1987). Although research activity in the areas of personality testing, modeling, and aggression has declined in recent years, the study of motivation; of anxiety, arousal, and performance; and of the group dynamics issues of social facilitation, leadership, and cohesion still remains popular (Landers et al., 1986). Motivation, especially from the attribution theory perspective, is the single most dominant area of research focus in sport psychology; publications and citations in this area far outweigh any other topic within the contemporary field (Landers et al., 1986a; LeUnes, Wolf, Ripper, & Anding, 1990). Recipient theories and paradigms from mainstream psychology (viz., the theories of attribution by Weiner, 1972; intrinsic motivation by Deci, 1975; self-efficacy by Bandura, 1977; competence motivation by Harter, 1978; and achievement motivation by Maehr & Nicholls, 1980) have dominated experimentation on motivation in the sport psychology field and are perhaps indicative of a more general failing of the field to (to date) develop many of its own theories despite the apparent need (see Dishman, 1983; Feltz, 1987). The development of a sport-specific measurement instrument for anxiety—Martens's (1977) Sport Competition Anxiety Test (SCAT)—has been in no small way responsible for the strong research activity on anxiety, arousal, and attention, although the use of self-report measures of all types remains a persistent source of controversy. Self-report measures such as Martens's

SCAT, Nideffer's (1976b) Test of Attentional and Interpersonal Style (TAIS), and McNair, Lorr, and Droppleman's (1971) Profile of Mood States (POMS) have been extremely popular with sport and exercise psychology researchers, although a number of influential researchers (e.g., Hatfield & Landers, 1983) have moved to psychophysiological methods in an attempt to overcome the limitations of self-report approaches. Given the multi-dimensional natures of most of the phenomena that sport and exercise psychology researchers seek to explain, the use of multiple levels of analysis to provide different vantage points to the phenomena of interest appears a desirable future direction for sport and exercise psychology research (Dishman, 1982) and indeed for all types of human action research (Stelmach, 1987).

New topics of research that emerged or blossomed in the sport and exercise psychology field in the 1980s were those related to performance enhancement and the use of various intervention strategies, to exercise and well-being, and to children and youth sport (Landers et al., 1986a). Concerns with performance enhancement have given rise to a whole new class of problem-driven research in which the emphasis is most frequently upon the psychological enhancement of the performances of individual athletes. This new research focus has been driven largely by the advent of a sport psychology profession and has been fueled substantially by two influential papers by Rainer Martens, the first advocating the use of more field-based research (Martens, 1979) and the second more radically advocating the use of more tacit sources of knowledge acquired by means other than application of the traditional methods of science (Martens, 1987). Although the emphases on ecological validity, on case studies, and on the understanding of individual differences are desirable ones, some researchers feel that any concerted applied research thrust should not be made without regard for theory development (Dishman, 1982; Gill, 1981; Harris, 1987; Landers, 1983). The advent of a sport psychology profession has led to a burgeoning development of new societies and new journals as well as some inevitable tensions regarding issues of registration, training, and the clinical-experimental mix. Current research interests on issues related to exercise and well-being represent a new focus on what is a very old question, although the broadening interest in issues such as exercise adherence (e.g., Dishman, 1988) draws the field closer to physiology and away from its traditional psychology parentage. The research emphasis on youth sport and, to a lesser extent, gender issues within contemporary sport and exercise psychology represent somewhat unique foci on particular populations of exercise participants. In the future we will probably see greater research attention given to some of the other significant subgroups within the sport environment about which relatively little is currently known (e.g., parents, officials, coaches/instructors, and the elderly).

Clearly, many of the issues with which the sport and exercise psychology field is grappling (e.g., ecological validity, application vs. theory, intrinsic vs. recipient theory development, multiple levels of analysis, and individual differences) are also issues of current relevance within the other human action fields. At a time when the sport and exercise psychology field is experiencing unprecedented popularity and growth, resolution of these issues by leading researchers in the field is crucial for the field's continued development.

The expert sport and exercise psychology researchers who contributed to this section have all made unique contributions to the development of knowledge in sport and exercise psychology, although they all have quite different perspectives on what are the crucial issues for the field and what theoretical perspectives and paradigms best progress understanding. Bert Carron, a former student of Franklin Henry, is a valuable link to the motor learning and control field, and although his research interests are now in the group dynamics area, trademark concerns with psychometric precision and vigor clearly remain evident in his work.

Bob Nideffer provides the archetypal example of the applied sport psychologist, and his TAIS instrument has proven a popular, albeit controversial, measure of attention, which has helped focus debate on the levels of analysis issue in sport psychology. Glyn Roberts operates clearly within a cognitive theoretical perspective; his work on attribution theory provides an excellent example of the importing, testing, and modifying of theories from mainstream psychology in the sport setting. In stark contrast, Brent Rushall advocates and experiments from within the behaviorist framework popularized in mainstream psychology by B.F. Skinner. The contrasts in the styles of all four experimenters are enlightening.

Chapter 10

Albert V. Carron

Faculty of Physical Education
University of Western Ontario
London, Ontario, Canada

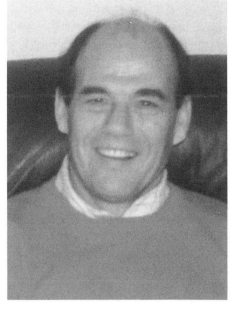

Bert Carron completed an undergraduate degree in physical education in 1963 from the University of Alberta in Edmonton, Canada, and followed this in 1965 with an MA degree from the same institution. He completed his doctorate, an EdD in educational psychology-physical education, 2 years later at the University of California at Berkeley under the supervision of Franklin Henry (see chapter 2). Immediately upon completing his graduate studies, Dr. Carron procured a teaching and research appointment in his native Canada in the School of Physical Education at the University of Saskatchewan in Saskatoon. The Saskatchewan appointment provided Carron with teaching experience in motor learning and control, research exposure to motor development (as part of the Saskatchewan Child Growth and Development Study headed by Professor Don Bailey), and an opportunity to coach in his favorite sport, American football. In 1974, Bert Carron accepted an associate professorship in the Faculty of Physical Education at the University of Western Ontario. He remains in the same department today, having been appointed a full professor in 1978.

Professor Carron has made significant contributions to all three areas of human action research. His contribution to motor learning and control has involved understanding the factors that selectively influence learning and performance, and his publications on fatigue effects, individual differences, and the generality/specificity issue (e.g., Carron, 1969c; Carron & Marteniuk, 1970; Leavitt & Carron, 1969) directly reflect the interests he developed during his graduate studies with Franklin Henry. His contributions to knowledge of age-related changes in motor performance arose largely from collaborative work with Don Bailey on the longitudinal database provided by the Saskatchewan Child Growth and Development Study (e.g., Carron & Bailey, 1973; Ellis, Carron, & Bailey, 1975), although he occasionally considered age as a mediating variable in some of his earlier motor learning and control work (e.g., Carron, 1971b). Having examined stress effects on motor performance as part of his master's thesis (e.g., Carron, 1968), Carron returned to a focus on sport psychology issues in the mid-1970s with his move to the faculty at Western Ontario. His early text *Social Psychology of Sport* (Carron, 1980) has been highly influential, as have subsequent texts on motivation (Carron, 1984) and group dynamics (Carron, 1988). As an experimenter in sport and exercise psychology, he is best known for his original contributions to knowledge in the group cohesion and leadership areas (arising largely from collaborative work with Chella Chelladurai, Larry Brawley, and Neil Widmeyer), although he has also contributed heavily to the motivation literature. Bert Carron has also maintained high-profile involvement in professional issues in the sport sciences in Canada and the United States, serving at various times and among other appointments as president of the Canadian Association of Sport Sciences and on the executive board of the Association for the Advancement of Applied Sport Psychology. He has served on the editorial board of the *Journal of Sport and Exercise Psychology* and as a section editor for the *Canadian Journal of Sport Sciences*.

In this chapter, Bert Carron chronicles the events leading to his transition in research focus from motor learning and control, to motor development, to his current focus on sport and exercise psychology, and he describes the parallel gradual transition from laboratory-based to field-based methods of inquiry. In reading this chapter remember that his path to research on sport and exercise psychology via a graduate education in motor learning and control is not atypical, because many of the researchers now prominent in sport and exercise psychology have reached the field in this way. For this reason, Carron's autobiographical chapter provides an excellent example of and personal insight into the career path of a contributor to the second emergence of the sport psychology field in North America. Carron's career and research direction, like those of many other researchers, have been influenced by an intricate weave of personal and situational influences, many of them beyond the experimenter's control or planning. His autobiography reveals how young researchers need not necessarily have grand research plans or fixed interests in order to successfully contribute to knowledge. Indeed, unplanned exposure to a range of different research fields and their methods may be of great benefit to a researcher. Like Jerry Thomas in chapter 9, Carron acknowledges the major role played by graduate students in innovative science, and the view Carron presents us of science as a social activity is important, and one that we consider in some detail in chapter 14.

AUTOBIOGRAPHY

"It all began in a little red schoolhouse in Edmonton, Alberta . . ."

My most difficult challenge in writing any article, chapter, or book has always been in developing the introduction. It's the foundation from which everything else flows, so it not only has to feel right but it has to effectively summarize the essence of the project. From my conversations with other writers I have found that this problem is, apparently, almost universal. In the early stages, their desk areas are also littered with piles of crumpled, discarded paper. This wasn't the case with this autobiography, however. In fact, the only difficulty I had was in choosing between two possible introductions. One of these, "It was a dark and stormy evening," was my early favorite. You might recognize this phrase, which has been immortalized by Snoopy, Charlie Brown's pet in the Charles Schultz cartoon *Peanuts*. Admittedly, it has absolutely no application to my career in sport psychology, but I liked it for two reasons. First, any phrase significant enough to launch a writing competition should be adequate to begin an autobiography.* Second, as B.F. Skinner (1956) observed, "some . . . parts of the scientific process do not now lend themselves to mathematical, logical, or any formal treatment" (p. 221). He's right, of course. My introduction into and journey through the field of sport psychology seems in retrospect to be marked by a series of random events. So, although the phrase "It was a dark and stormy evening" may seem illogical as an introduction to an autobiography, that very quality is what initially appealed to me. At any rate, at my editor's insistence I abandoned it.

The one I like is "It all began in a little red schoolhouse in Edmonton, Alberta." It has some appealing advantages. First, it's the type of phrase

---

*"It was a dark and stormy night" was originally used by Edward Bulwer-Lytton to introduce one of his works. Scott Rice, of San Jose State University, initiated a writing competition in which it is mandatory that authors begin their stories with this Bulwer-Lytton line (e.g., Rice, 1984).

that should be included in every biography. And, unlike, "It was a dark and stormy evening," it's partly true. I did go to school in Edmonton. And some of the buildings where I attended classes in elementary, junior high, and high school, and at the University of Alberta (where I obtained my undergraduate degree and then a master's degree in physical education), were red in color. But I also should point out that although this phrase is close to the truth, it's not the total truth. My initiation into the field of physical education and sport psychology is probably more closely associated with little red schoolhouses in places like Windsor and Australia and California. The schoolhouses in these locations were instrumental in the development of teachers who subsequently played significant roles in my academic development, who counseled me to enter physical education and/or supervised my initial work in sport psychology. Take Windsor, for example. Gino Fracas, my high school physical education teacher and coach (later he was also one of my teachers and coaches at the University of Alberta, and most recently he is a professional colleague) attended school there. Gino is an outstanding role model as an educator and a person and was probably the primary reason I decided to enter physical education. A secondary reason was that I wanted to work in counseling psychology (although I didn't know it by that name when I was 18 years old). High school teaching in general and physical education specifically seemed like the best avenues for me to achieve that purpose. So, an interest in teaching, an interest in sport, and an interest in counseling were the origins of my interest in sport psychology.

The fact that I ultimately satisfied my sport psychology interests at the university level rather than through teaching and coaching in high school is probably associated with a red schoolhouse in Australia, Max Howell's native country. When I was an undergraduate student at the University of Alberta, Max was the director of graduate affairs. The University of Alberta had recently developed a graduate program that was to become among the largest in North America. The program was achieving an international flavor as students were recruited from all over the world. As an undergraduate student I was aware of this. Also, I did find the science courses in physical education and my options in psychology challenging and interesting. So after a number of discussions with Max, I finally decided to enter the graduate program and specialize in the area of sport psychology.

The red schoolhouse in California is the University of California in Berkeley, where Max Howell and Bob Morford (the latter my master's thesis adviser) both obtained their doctorate degrees. Bob and Max were the catalysts for my decision to go on to doctoral work with their thesis adviser, Franklin Henry. The decision to study with Franklin was one I've never regretted—even when I was hopping over the hot coals that are a part of every graduate student's journey. It was an intensive program, although in retrospect the essence of the program was an apprenticeship with Franklin. In every other respect—course requirements, comprehensive exams, difficulty, and challenges—it was undoubtedly similar to most other doctoral programs. Franklin Henry made the difference. In addition to his seminars, which were taught every semester, he met with us daily—noontime brown-bag seminars 7 days a week. And, those informal sessions often became heated. In response to my questions about a noontime session I didn't attend, a fellow graduate student told me, "Nothing out of the ordinary happened; there were two suicides and a mental breakdown." As a writer and editor, Franklin was without equal. His infamous phrase, "words have meaning," which he generally used prior to wielding his editorial red pen, continues to awaken former students in the dead of night in cold sweats. The writing of a dissertation was a step-by-step process, with Franklin changing words, sentences, and paragraphs, page by page. After graduation, I met another former doctoral student who said, "I read your thesis, Bert; Franklin did his usual great job of writing." No further explanations were necessary. No questions were asked. We'd both been there; we knew. It has been over 25 years since I left Berkeley, and I have yet to meet a scientist more thorough, knowledgeable, brilliant, and demanding of his students and himself than Franklin.

So, if all began in a little red schoolhouse insofar as my research interests are concerned, the one in Berkeley was perhaps the most influential. Obviously, there continue to be other influences. Skinner (1956), commenting about his development as a scientist, noted that "the scientist, like any organism, is the product of a unique history" (p. 233). It's true, of course. What I know and do today are products of Alberta, Berkeley, and other experiences both direct and indirect: contacts with teachers and scientists, with research collaborators, with undergraduate and graduate students, and with the research and scholarship of others. Those experiences have been the significant factors in any research in which I've been involved. It would be nice to look back and say that I've always had a giant plan for my research; a quest to describe, explain, and ultimately predict sport and physical activity behavior; a drive to develop the sport psychology equivalent of Hullian-Spence drive theory (given that Hullian-Spence drive theory is currently in disfavor, the wonder of it all is that I didn't succeed in this line). But, I simply didn't have such a plan. I read the research of others, listened to their papers, discussed ideas, and from this foundation developed research ideas either alone or in collaboration.

I can best illustrate the roles and importance of significant others in my research efforts by examining the various problem areas I've investigated. Although there have been some minor exceptions, four general issues have held my interests at various times in my professional life: the analysis of factors influencing skill acquisition; the study of the relative importance of inter- and intra–individual differences to motor performance; the examination of parameters influencing human growth and development;

and the study of group dynamics including interpersonal compatibility, leadership, and group cohesion. In order to illustrate the roles that others have had in this research, I'd like to discuss how I became interested in each of these areas.

My initial interests (which I pursued in my master's thesis) concerned the effects that anxiety and stress have on motor performance and learning (Carron, 1968; Carron & Morford, 1968). Like all research, this study evolved from the work of others. Janet Taylor had published her personality test, the Manifest Anxiety Scale (MAS) (Taylor, 1953), and numerous researchers in psychology were using it as a measure of drive to test predictions emanating from Hullian-Spence drive theory. The MAS and that general line of research appealed to me. Also, anyone working in the area of learning quickly becomes familiar with Tolman's classic work in the area of latent learning (Tolman, 1932). Tolman observed that reinforcement (or reward) directly influences performance but not learning. Tolman's early work was done with rats, but the general applicability of his proposition for human learning also intrigued me. So the idea for my master's thesis evolved from the work in psychology associated with Taylor's anxiety measure, Hullian-Spence drive theory, and Tolman's work on latent learning.

For the thesis, I tested the total university freshman population on the MAS (this was back in the good old days when John Loy was in his early 40s and compulsory physical education existed for all 1st-year students). I selected individuals at the two extremes and introduced electric shock as a stressor during practice on a motor task, the stabilometer. What I remember most vividly was the time required to test 120 individuals over 2 days, 35 trials a day. It seemed like my life was passing in front of me in the test room. I later used a similar experimental design in my doctoral dissertation. So, if the phrase "Fool me once, shame on you: fool me twice, shame on me" has any validity, the only conclusion to be drawn about my early experimental design decisions is "shame on me." There's absolutely no sense getting older if you don't get smarter, so I'm now working on smarter. I hire research assistants and/or use shorter test sessions.

Although it's not chronological, I should note that my interest in the factors that influence performance versus learning continued after I completed my doctorate. A number of Franklin Henry's students had pursued dissertations examining the influence of physical warm-up on performance. During my doctoral program I reviewed this literature for Franklin's course in physiology of exercise. A knowledge of that literature, coupled with the influence of Tolman's classic work, was also the basis for a series of studies I was involved with concerning the effects of fatigue on motor learning and performance (e.g., Carron, 1969c).

My doctoral dissertation (Carron, 1969a, 1969b) and a number of projects that Jack Leavitt and I undertook on the effect of practice on inter- and intra–individual differences (e.g., Carron & Leavitt, 1968a, 1968b) evolved directly from discussions and graduate experiences with Franklin Henry. Franklin had written a short article in which he fractionated total variance into true score variance, intravariance, and error (Henry, 1959). It was a general topic and methodology with which his graduate students became very familiar, and frequently dissertations resulted, including my own. The independent projects with Jack resulted from the brainstorming sessions so prevalent in any good graduate program. Those projects gave us confidence in our abilities to develop, carry out, and report on research projects on our own. We also learned a variety of other things, including the difference between reality and the ivory tower. For example, I recall some testing we carried out in core area schools in the city of Oakland. We intended to test a group of adolescent males on both the stabilometer and the pursuit rotor. We set up our equipment in different rooms and began testing subjects. At the end of the morning, we compared experiences. My subjects had rhythmically gyrated to the music from the oversized radios they carried—while balancing on the stabilometer. Jack's tracking test had been converted into a fencing task—to music. It never occurred to us to try to describe, explain, or predict the subjects' behavior, the failure to comply with our experimental instructions. We were too busy being scientists. So, we packed our equipment and left.

My first job following the completion of my doctorate in 1967 was at the University of Saskatchewan in Saskatoon. Part of my responsibility was to teach motor learning at the undergraduate and graduate levels. I was also an assistant football coach with the university team. This latter responsibility led to what must rate as a one-of-a-kind experience. The head coach, Dan Marisi, was also enrolled in the graduate program in physical education, and I was his thesis adviser. So, he was my supervisor, and I was his supervisor. We quickly reached a compromise solution; I was responsible for confusing him in motor learning; he was responsible for confusing me in football. Independent raters have never been able to reach consensus on who was more successful.

At Saskatchewan, I published my first book, a lab manual in motor learning (Carron, 1971a) and continued to carry out research in this area. But I slowly became assimilated into the Saskatchewan Child Growth and Development Study, a 10-year longitudinal study designed to assess parameters associated with the impact of physical activity on the physical growth of children. Although that assimilation was gradual, in hindsight it was probably quite inevitable. The chief investigator, Don Bailey, was intelligent, creative, and knowledgeable about his area and the gaps in understanding that existed within it. Like those of any good teacher, his ideas and work were stimulating and interesting. My interests gradually developed from our discussions, and subsequently we collaborated on some projects (e.g., Carron & Bailey, 1974). I believe that if I had stayed at Saskatchewan, I would now be working almost exclusively in child growth and development. Ideas for research were plentiful, and there was considerable data analyses and writing to be done. But, in 1973 the University of Western Ontario was looking for a replacement for Terry Orlick in sport psychology. When I was offered the position, I accepted.*

My transition from motor learning to growth and development to sport psychology was most heavily influenced by situational factors. This is not to suggest that personal dispositions and preferences had no influence. My initial interests in motor learning had always been on macrophenomena such as stress, anxiety, fatigue, and individual differences. As research in motor learning within physical education and kinesiology evolved, the use of information-processing models became more prevalent. Behaviors that took place in milliseconds became the focus in research, and I couldn't generate any enthusiasm for what were the pertinent issues. My natural interests were in the content of sport psychology (including the relatively more macrovariables of stress, anxiety, personality, leadership, cognitions, and motivation), so my reading, writing, and research simply shifted slightly. But, there is no doubt that situational factors were critical to my entry into sport psychology. And, the move from Saskatchewan was the most important.

My research at the University of Western Ontario has focused on the area of group dynamics, although I have written in the general area of sport psychology (Carron, 1980, 1981, 1984). Again, the role of others has been important. For example, one of the areas in which I've carried out research with colleagues and graduate students is interpersonal compatibility (e.g., Carron & Bennett, 1977). My introduction to this area came when a graduate student, Liz Johnston, prepared a term paper that included a discussion of William Schutz's (1966) book, *The Interpersonal Underworld*, and his measure of interpersonal compatibility, Fundamental Interpersonal Relations Orientation—Behavior (FIRO-B) (Schutz, 1967). At that time there had been a considerable amount of discussion in popular and scientific writing about the authoritarian nature of athletic coaches and how this personality type was incompatible with the needs of athletes. I intuitively felt that this didn't make sense. Because compatibility and incompatibility are social constructs, it seemed logical that the needs of both individuals in the dyad (the coach and the athlete) are critical. Schutz's model and inventory provided a means to evaluate this issue.

My work with Chella Chelladurai is another example of the role that others have played in my development. Chella, my colleague at Western, is interested in the management science of sport and physical activity. The parallels between the research in management science and sport psychology are considerable. The two general areas share an interest in the most common and critical measures of group effectiveness—

---

*Terry has pointed out to me that when he left Western, the university had to hire two people in sport psychology to replace him, Bonnie Bennett and me.

individual and group productivity and satisfaction. The areas also share a number of correlates of productivity and satisfaction including group cohesion, leadership, and group norms and roles. As a consequence of the overlap between our areas of interest and our personal compatibility, Chella and I collaborated on a number of projects in leadership (e.g., Chelladurai & Carron, 1978) and cohesion (e.g., Carron & Chelladurai, 1981).

My current research focus has been in the area of group cohesion. My initiation into this area is interesting because it highlights the role that good graduate students can play in their professors' development. People unfamiliar with graduate student research often assume that the teacher teaches and the student learns. With good students, however, the learning process goes in two directions; both teach and learn. This was the case with Jim Ball, a graduate student who came to me with an idea for research in group cohesion. At that time, I hadn't done any research in this area and was only marginally familiar with the literature. Through constant discussions and reading, we developed a research problem involving the assessment of cohesion, participation motivation, and performance of ice hockey teams throughout an intercollegiate season. Subsequently, we obtained a grant that helped us complete the research, and the results were published (Ball & Carron, 1976). Jim's insights as well as the insights I picked up during the project sufficiently stimulated my interest to the extent that I've continued in this line of research.

Presently, my research in cohesiveness is so completely collaborative with Larry Brawley and Neil Widmeyer of the University of Waterloo that it's impossible to present a personal—as opposed to a group—perspective (e.g., Brawley, Carron, & Widmeyer, 1987; Carron, Widmeyer, & Brawley, 1985; Widmeyer, Brawley, & Carron, 1985). The three of us began working together in 1981. That year Neil went on sabbatical, and I was approached by Waterloo to teach his undergraduate class. I commuted to Waterloo once a week, and met with Larry and Neil (who had remained in Waterloo during his leave) prior to the class to discuss selected topics in sport psychology. We shared an interest in group dynamics, so it was obviously one of the issues that surfaced repeatedly. Also, coincidentally, that year I was invited to present a keynote address at the annual meeting of the North American Society for the Psychology of Sport and Physical Activity. My topic was centered on group dynamics generally and group cohesiveness specifically (Carron, 1981, 1982). Larry and Neil provided me with numerous reactions to the paper. One conclusion that seemed to jump out at us was that there was a need to develop a psychometrically sound instrument to assess cohesiveness in sport teams. The three of us and Chella Chelladurai applied for a grant and undertook the project. Unfortunately, Chella had to leave the group after a year due to other commitments. The remaining three of us have continued to meet approximately twice a month over the last 10 years. Like every effective group, we bring different strengths and assume different complementary roles. Neil summarized this latter point best when he observed, "For every Martha there has to be a Mary." So like every effective group, we try to systematically rotate the Martha and Mary roles.*

Initially, I pointed out that my most difficult challenge in writing any article, chapter, or book has been in developing the introduction. The second most difficult challenge is the conclusion. As was the case with the introduction, settling on a conclusion wasn't overly difficult here. Again, the only difficulty I had was in choosing between two possibilities. One that seems appropriate is represented by a line in Alfred Tennyson's poem *Ulysses*: "I am a part of all that I have met." No researcher starts, grows, or proceeds in a vacuum. Science is a social activity, and without the foundation provided by the thoughts, research, and writing of others, it would stagnate and die. I hope the extent of my indebtedness to others has come through in this autobiography.

Another conclusion that is also appropriate is best summed up by the comments of a friend when I told her I was invited to write an autobiographical chapter. Her immediate reaction was, "Who would be interested in that?" Who indeed? Notwithstanding the fact that prophets (and physical educators) are sometimes without honor in their own homes, she does have a point.

---

*Readers of the Bible will be familiar with the story of Martha and Mary, Lazarus's sisters. They were friends of Jesus, and Martha, the older, was the mistress of the house. During a visit from Jesus, she assumed responsibility for the preparation of the meal, while Mary sat at his feet and listened. When Martha complained about Mary's lack of help in the kitchen, Jesus pointed out that people have different roles to play and that Mary's role was not only necessary, it was the more important.

Chapter 11

Robert M. Nideffer

Enhanced Performance Systems
San Diego, California, U.S.A.

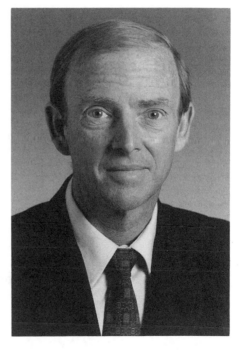

Robert Nideffer was born in Oxnard, California, in 1942. A collegiate diver and the holder of a black belt in aikido, he formalized his practical interest in sport psychology with studies in the clinical psychology field. He obtained his undergraduate science degree in psychology from Lewis and Clark College in Portland, Oregon, in 1967 and followed this with an MA in psychology from Vanderbilt University in Nashville, Tennessee, 2 years later. Nideffer completed a PhD in clinical and experimental psychology at Vanderbilt in 1971 and the same year began a teaching and research position as an assistant professor in the Department of Psychology and Psychiatry at the University of Rochester in the state of New York. Dr. Nideffer remained at Rochester until 1977, when he assumed a position of professor at the California School of Professional Psychology in San Diego, a position he retained until 1983. In 1977 Dr. Nideffer founded a private company, Enhanced Performance Systems, as an outlet for his training programs and materials for sport, business, education, and the military. He is president of that organization today on a full-time basis, although he retains some links to the tertiary education sector through a part-time teaching appointment in the Department of Physical Education at San Diego State University. He is a current editorial board member of *The Sport Psychologist*.

As an experimenter, Bob Nideffer is best known for his development of the Test of Attentional and Interpersonal Style (TAIS) (Nideffer, 1976b), a pencil-and-paper test designed to assess an individual's strengths and weaknesses with respect to the strategic allocation of attention to particular sport or work tasks. The TAIS has been used substantially as a research tool, although it has not been without its critics (e.g., Dewey, Brawley, & Allard, 1989; Summers & Ford, 1990). Specific questions about the psychometrics of the TAIS have helped to focus more fruitful debate within the sport and exercise psychology field upon the general utility of self-report methods and upon the best approaches for experimenters to use in tackling multidimensional problems posed by ubiquitous phenomena such as attention. Robert Nideffer's contributions to the sport and exercise psychology field have been particularly valued by clinical psychologists working on a one-to-one basis with athletes in the field, and his lay-level texts, *The Inner Athlete* (Nideffer, 1976a) and *A.C.T.: Attention Control Training* (Nideffer & Sharpe, 1978), have been extremely popular at the grass-roots level. Nideffer has also written extensively on clinical issues and issues related to the profession (in particular, his 1981 *Ethics and Practice of Applied Sport Psychology* has been widely read), and he has written on mental practice (e.g., Nideffer, 1987a) and on the psychology of the injured athlete (e.g., Nideffer, 1983). The prevailing themes throughout his writing focus on the structuring of attention and concentration and on their assessment and improvement. These are familiar topics to most students in the applied sport psychology field.

Nideffer is unique among our assembled expert experimenters in terms of his training: clinical psychology rather than kinesiology/physical education. He makes this clinical orientation clear in his chapter, particularly where he discusses his approach to research. Note, in reading his autobiographical contribution, his preoccupation with the problem-solving aspects of science and the excitement he generates out of this and out of the writing process. Nideffer's comments on the need for a balance between basic and applied research are also important, as is his reasoning that applied research is most enjoyable because it impounds directly on day-to-day living.

AUTOBIOGRAPHY

It will be interesting to me to read the chapters other authors have contributed to this book, because I have never considered myself a "real" experimenter. In my mind, real experimenters are much more self-disciplined than I am. Real experimenters are more singled minded (more narrowly focused). Real experimenters are scholars; they know the literature inside out and spend hours each day in their laboratories and/or in libraries. Real experimenters polish their products and take the risks of rejection by applying for grants. I greatly respect and admire real experimenters, but if my definition is accurate, I could never be one.

I graduated from high school with a 1.8 grade-point average on a 4.0 scale. The highest grade I received in an English class was a D. I flunked speech in the 11th grade because I was afraid to stand up in front of the class. I flunked study hall because I wouldn't study. I had no self-discipline, and I wouldn't give in to any structure that others attempted to impose on me. The only thing that I did to distinguish myself was get arrested in the 9th grade for setting a bomb off under the main street of town. If they had given grades for rebelling, I would have earned an A.

To the outside viewer, it may appear as if things have changed. I did go to college and graduate school. I was disciplined enough to earn a PhD in clinical and experimental psychology at Vanderbilt. Over the past 15 years I have written 10 books and authored around 100 papers. In spite of these outward trappings, I don't fit the model I just outlined. I am so busy doing my own thing that I spend little time reading the works of others, a fact I often feel guilty about. I have refused to follow traditional academic routes, in part because I have been afraid of rejection and failure. I have been so sensitive to criticism that I once placed a rejected article in a desk drawer for a month before I could look at the reviewer's comments.

In spite of the rather negative self-evaluation I just presented, I have had fun. Like Frank Sinatra, I have managed to be successful by doing it my way. I believe very strongly that there is a place for the traditional researcher and a place for people like me. The research in which I have engaged has been tremendously exciting. I wouldn't change places with anyone!

Developing a Commitment

I spent 3 years in the U.S. Army right after I completed high school. This was an important period in my life; I gained a little self-discipline, but more importantly I developed the interest that became the focal point of my career. It was an interest that motivated me to make the long-term commitment to earn a PhD and develop a research program.

While in the army, I spent 2 years in Japan, during which time I studied the martial arts of aikido and karate. These two disciplines emphasized the fact that physical performance was to a great extent dependent upon psychological factors. Time and time again I saw my instructor perform at a level and under conditions that were well beyond normal bounds. I left the service determined to get into college: I wanted to explore the role of psychological variables in human performance.

I wanted to be able to understand, control, and predict behavior (my own and others). I hoped to find relationships that would generalize from person to person. Although at the time I couldn't articulate it, I wanted to develop my own theory of human behavior, a theory that would explain the full range of human performance from supernormal behavior to psychotic behavior.

I felt a strong need to be of service to others, and I believed the best way I could serve people would be to help them maximize their own potential. My goal to increase our ability to understand, predict, and control human behavior was total.

Let me define *total* for you. I have good analytical skills, and I am very introspective. I examine anything that I observe or learn to see what it can contribute to my goal. Intuitively, I continually employ the scientific method. I make observations and then use these observations to make predictions about behavior. When it's possible, I will create conditions formally or informally (i.e., experiment) to test my assumptions. Then I will observe the results and modify my hypotheses. That process is as natural to me as breathing.

Total commitment also means I am stubborn and selfish. Others can control me only as long as that control facilitates my goal of increasing my (and their) ability to understand, predict, and control behavior. When I don't feel as if I am making progress along these lines, I drop out. As you might imagine, my behavior can place an incredible amount of pressure on those people who work with me, since I expect the same commitment from them.

College

Without a great deal of luck, I never would have developed a research program. An individual's personality characteristics are neither good nor bad; depending upon situational factors they become assets or liabilities. Although my goal might be to recognize my own characteristics and to consciously match my abilities to the demands of the environment, there are times when that is impossible. I have been very lucky through my career. I was lucky to find colleges and professors that either indulged my weaknesses or compensated for them.

It was blind luck that caused me to choose a small liberal arts college in the Pacific Northwest. If that school had not encouraged me to think for myself, and had not tolerated my poor spelling and punctuation, I would not have survived the education system. At Lewis and Clark College, personal enthusiasm and the content of the things that I had to say were more important than the form. I was evaluated on the basis of my ability to relate material to my own life and to the lives of others. As far as I was concerned I was in heaven.

It was at Lewis and Clark that I began doing research. It was at Lewis and Clark that I learned about the scientific method, finding a label for my own thought processes. It was at Lewis and Clark that I discovered the importance of putting my thoughts down on paper and of subjecting them to a formal or public test. At Lewis and Clark I was rewarded for engaging in the process of research, not for the outcome of the study. It was easy to take risks when all I had to do was play the game to win. The results of the study were the icing on the cake.

Graduate School

At Vanderbilt, I was confronted with the fact that my life at Lewis and Clark had been a little like living in the Garden of Eden. I was reminded that success according to my academic peers depended upon outcome as well as process. Academic position, financial support through grants, and publications all depended upon significant results. How I played the game was no longer enough.

My first year in graduate school was almost a disaster. During that year we studied the core areas of psychology. We were expected to accumulate a great deal of information and to then feed the information back on tests. There was no time for thinking and relating the material to other areas. It was high school all over again. I survived that year for two reasons. First, I did work hard because I knew that I wanted the education; I could see past the 1st year. Although I worked hard, it was difficult for me to study on others' terms. My grades were .1 point below what the department required. Second, I was saved because my research adviser saw promise. Like my professors at Lewis and Clark, my research adviser valued my ability to think in an integrative way, to relate new material to previous experience. Without Dr. Rue Cromwell's support, I would have been dropped from the graduate program.

The constant reminder that we were being evaluated created a number of problems for students. It was easy to become overwhelmed by the demands of the educational process. The feeling that we had to know everything paralyzed some students and kept them from performing. They couldn't bring themselves to complete their research until they were sure they knew everything.

Often students lost interest in research because they felt they had to compromise their ideas. They felt they had to sterilize projects so much in order to make them defensible that the projects lost their value. Other students tried to get faculty to define research projects for them. In this way they reduced the anxiety of having their own ideas evaluated.

Unfortunately, when the ideas weren't their own, the students found it difficult to maintain the level of motivation necessary to complete and defend the work.

I was spared these problems, largely because of my research adviser. At Vanderbilt, a graduate student in psychology was expected to have a research adviser within the first 8 weeks of the 1st year. As you might expect, this resulted in students searching frantically for anybody they thought they might be able to work with. Once again, I lucked out. I asked Dr. Cromwell to supervise my research because he was one of the few faculty members engaged in research that related to more complex human behaviors.

Dr. Cromwell was interested in studying attentional processes in schizophrenia. I admired him. His strategy with a student who wanted to work with him was to describe his line of research and show the student how the studies going on within the department of psychiatry fit into a total program. This made it possible for me to see that what I previously thought was meaningless laboratory research really had some value. Dr. Cromwell showed me that you could, and should, look beyond your data. That is not to say that you draw conclusions based on speculations; rather you use speculation to motivate yourself and to begin to generate testable hypotheses. He continually reminded me of the importance of being able to relate my research to the world, no matter how basic that research was.

Dr. Cromwell did not tell his students what they should study; he expected them to come up with studies that fit in with the total program. He relied on students and staff to develop research ideas that he then helped them refine. I couldn't have found a more perfect situation. I was allowed to be creative, and at the same time I had someone who would "pick up" after me and who would provide me with the structure I needed. It was Dr. Cromwell who taught me how to organize my writing. He tried to get me to improve my spelling and punctuation, but he couldn't have everything.

Dr. Cromwell appreciated my enthusiasm, and because of that, I think, he tolerated the fact that I tended to strip the things that I needed to learn to the bare essentials. Unlike some of the other students, I didn't become overwhelmed with all I had to learn. If I was working on a particular project, I would very carefully map out the skills that I needed and I would develop these, but I wouldn't learn any more than I needed at the time. I am sure, for example, that Dr. Cromwell would have liked me to know more about statistics in general. Instead, I developed a very thorough understanding of those statistics I used and let my knowledge of other techniques slide.

Dr. Cromwell helped me strike a balance between basic laboratory research and more directly applied studies. He encouraged my attempts to apply the things I was learning about attention to sports; at the same time he emphasized the importance of scientifically testing what I was doing. He also showed me how important it was to be close to my data.

I learned that research is much like psychological assessment. The researcher's ability to explain what happened in the study depends upon his or her being close to every aspect of that study. Research on human subjects is too complex and is affected by too many uncontrolled variables. To be a good researcher you must be a sensitive observer of your subjects and your experimental procedures. A major source of my enthusiasm for the things I have done has been the fact that I have been intimately involved in every aspect of the study.

Although my research in graduate school was fairly narrowly defined laboratory experimentation, I was relating it to virtually every aspect of my life. I was continually asking myself what the behavior of schizophrenic patients said about my behavior, or that of my aikido instructor. Likewise, when I had to learn a skill, I first thought about how I might integrate what I was learning with my desire to further understand, predict, and control behavior. How could I use statistics, computers, electroencephalograms, biofeedback, and assessment techniques in the development of my theory?

Publish or Perish

The pressure to publish or perish has created problems for a lot of researchers. I am sure that if I had given into that pressure and allowed it to dictate my activity, I would have been much less productive. I know that when I write because I want to, the reviews are much better than when I write because I feel I have to.

The joy of experimentation, as far as I am concerned, is the detective work or problem solving that is involved. Hypotheses are generated from observations; these hypotheses develop out of introspection. The challenge to get inside of myself, to ask questions, and to attempt to understand something I have observed is exciting. Being creative and developing ways of putting those hypotheses to the test are also exciting. Then, independent of the outcome, the real joy occurs when I feel I am able to explain why my original hypotheses were correct or incorrect.

When I am writing or doing research to please myself, I am rewarded whether the results meet a journal editor's criteria for publication or not. There is a great deal to be learned independent of the outcome! I believe that some of the best things I have ever written will never be published. Those were articles or books that involved a great deal of introspection and detective work. Often, the problem was so complex that it would take a lifetime of studies or a new, as yet undeveloped, research methodology to test the ideas.

By writing for myself, I have avoided the pressure that comes with the academic demand to publish or perish. I write to clarify and to express my thoughts and ideas. Writing itself is a part of the detective process. Writing is something that I enjoy, and something I would do, independent of academia.

Clinical Assessment Versus Experimental Research

It has always seemed ironic to me that the mode number of publications for PhD's in clinical psychology is one! That one publication is more often than not the individual's doctoral dissertation. The good clinical psychologist is an excellent experimentalist. The good clinical psychologist uses the scientific method to understand, predict, and control complex human behavior. In spite of this fact, most clinical psychologists do not consider themselves researchers.

Clinicians pride themselves on their instincts, their intuitions, and their abilities to listen with a third ear. Great athletes and successful business executives alike respond to their instincts or "gut feelings." To me, words like *instinct* and *intuition* are words you use to describe the fact that you have been successful without knowing what you were reading and reacting to. The sixth sense is little more than paying attention to the right cues, identifying the signal in all of the noise around you. Just because you can't immediately articulate what you reacted to doesn't mean there aren't lawful relationships to be discovered.

When I left graduate school, I accepted a position as an assistant professor in the Department of Psychology at the University of Rochester. I was hired to conduct research, to supervise the research of graduate students, and to teach psychological assessment skills to clinical students.

The focus of my own research developed out of my desire to improve the assessment skills of the students I was training. Some of the assessment techniques the students were using seemed to encourage intellectual and artistic creativity independent of any predictive validity. For example, students might become very creative with their interpretations of a subject's responses to ink blots. Although interesting and of literary merit, their interpretations didn't help develop treatment plans or increase the predictability of the client's behavior.

At the other extreme were instruments like the Minnesota Multiphasic Personality Inventory (MMPI) that encouraged the students to suspend their own judgment and creativity and instead to accept a prognosis or diagnosis based on its previous statistical frequency. Students using such instruments often ignored critical situational and individual differences in favor of placing responsibility for conclusions on a cookbook.

I felt I could get a great deal of very useful information out of a Rorschach Ink Blot Test or an MMPI. My experience and my use of the experimental method led me to develop hypotheses about responses, to make predictions based on the hypotheses, to then examine patient behavior (through the interview and/or past history), and to validate or to invalidate and revise my opinions. As a function of that thinking process, I could make my own judgments about the relevance and validity of test information.

I found that my students too attempted to use the experimental method, albeit informally. These were bright analytical individuals. They were using the right method, but somehow they weren't seeing the right things (collecting the right data). Questions that I began asking myself were very personal. How could a student and I look at the same data and come up with very different interpretations? What was I seeing that made me a much better predictor of patient behavior than the students I was teaching?

I believe that each of us, to survive, develops an implicit if not explicit set of constructs that we use to help us understand our world and to predict behavior. Highly successful individuals are those with the best set of constructs for their particular situations. Somewhat egotistical, I felt I had a pretty good set of constructs for predicting behavior across a wide variety of situations. I felt that I could help my students by sharing my constructs or theory. My theory would teach them what to observe, what to look for in performance situations. The students would then use their analytical skills and abilities to test the data that they collected to see if it would enhance their abilities to understand, predict, and (if desired) control the client.

Developing the Test of Attentional and Interpersonal Style

One of the things that has allowed me to enjoy my work has been the fact that I don't think too far ahead. I know that if I anticipate all of the work needed to develop and validate a test, I probably won't even begin the process. I just take things one step at a time; each step is an end goal in itself. This means I am rewarded at virtually every stage of the process.

The first thing I did in developing an assessment tool for my students was attempt to identify those cues I was reading that helped me anticipate and/or explain behavior. To help myself and to help the students I had to identify cues that were operative across people and across situations. Without some generalizability, there was no way to predict from one situation to the next. Because I had ample evidence to suggest that I was quite successful in predicting across situations, I knew lawful relationships existed; I just had to discover them. I began by analyzing my own behavior and the aspects of my behavior that seemed consistent across situations. Having done that, I looked to see if the things I saw in myself fit other people as well.

My initial analysis led to the identification of several attentional (concentration) and interpersonal characteristics that I felt were "transsituational." These were things like the ability to think analytically, the need to be in control of interpersonal situations, and the ability and/or willingness to express anger.

Once I identified these performance-relevant characteristics, I had to operationally or behaviorally define them. For example, criticizing an instructor in front of a class is a behavioral example of expressing anger and of taking control of a situation. Depending upon the nature of the criticism (e.g., logical vs. emotional), it might also provide behavioral evidence of good analytical skills.

In my assessment classes, I began pointing out to students behavioral examples of the particular attentional and interpersonal characteristics I was reading that helped me understand their patients. Students found this useful, and the next logical step was to develop an instrument that measured these characteristics directly so the students did not have to intuitively separate them from other sources of data.

To do this, I listed behaviorally focused items that I believed provided evidence of the behaviors or skills I was trying to measure. At the time I was writing the items, I was not worried about establishing validity for the test or publishing what I was doing. I was not engaged in research, so I could publish a paper.

When I started this project, my intent was to create an assessment tool my students and I could use, something I hoped we would find useful in predicting patient behavior and in providing directions for counseling and/or training.

I realized that to create the instrument, I needed to develop some normative data, to demonstrate the reliability of the test's subscales, and to establish some type of test-retest reliability. This was a relatively simple process. The rewards for doing it were the correlations that resulted. There was some internal consistency, the subscales were independent, and there was good test-retest reliability.

There were other rewards too. The first version of the test attempted to measure four different types of concentration or attentional focuses. Statistical analyses indicated we were measuring only three. I wasn't rewarded through confirmation of what I wanted to do; instead, I was rewarded by being presented with another problem to solve. Why didn't I have four types of attention? Was my hypothesis wrong? Was something wrong with the items?

The Test of Attentional and Interpersonal Style has helped me articulate my own theory of human behavior. Current research allows me to attempt to validate the utility of the instrument and my theory. I win no matter what the outcome of the research. If results are as I expect, they provide some support for my ideas. If results are not as I expect, they force me to problem solve, to revise my thoughts, and ultimately to improve my ability to understand, predict, and control behavior.

Summary

One of the purposes of this book is to show students that research can be fun. In summary, I would like to highlight those factors that make research fun for me.

Most importantly, the research in which I have engaged has had very real meaning for my life. My research has not been narrowly focused; instead it has had tremendous generalizability. I have studied attentional and interpersonal skills that are directly related to performance in virtually every aspect of life. The things I learn can be applied at home, at the office, on the playing field, at school, or at war. Because I have had something to gain that is independent of the results of the research, I have not been paralyzed by concerns over outcome or the need to publish. The process of research has been personally or intrinsically rewarding.

I wrote the 1976 article that described the development and validation of the Test of Attentional and Interpersonal Style as an afterthought. I did not begin the research with the idea of publishing. Invariably, my best writing and research has occurred when the only pressure to produce has come from within!

As others have become interested in and used my theory, I have been extrinsically rewarded. I have been rewarded for outcome, but that has been the icing on the cake. I have been highly productive without trying. I haven't had to make myself go to the laboratory. Life is my laboratory, and that is something I enjoy being intimately involved with

My research and writing have allowed me to travel all over the world. I have been able to work with people who perform at all levels: Olympic and professional athletes, highly trained military personnel, business executives, health care workers, and psychiatric patients.

As I mentioned at the outset, I have been lucky. I have been involved with people who have accepted and/or compensated for my weaknesses. I have been supported by professors, students, family, and friends. I haven't had any more talent or ability than most people. My stubbornness has been an asset most of the time, and in spite of my sensitivity to rejection I have been willing to take some risks. I think the real key to my own success, however, has been that I haven't looked too far ahead. I have become caught up in the process of research and have largely ignored or been unconcerned with outcome.

Chapter 12

Glyn C. Roberts

Department of Kinesiology
University of Illinois at Urbana-Champaign
Urbana-Champaign, Illinois, U.S.A.

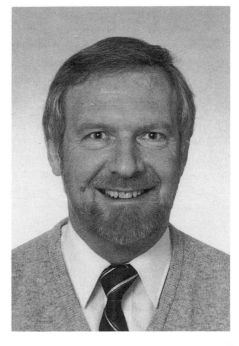

Glyn Roberts was born in Cheshire, England, in 1940. He completed a certificate of education at Loughborough College in 1961 before assuming a position as head of physical education and head coach of soccer and track and field at City of Coventry Boarding School. In 1965, Roberts emigrated to the United States, furthering his education with a master's degree from the University of Massachusetts in 1966 (with a major in physical education and a minor in history) and a PhD from the University of Illinois in 1969 (with a major in physical education and a minor in social psychology). Upon completing his doctorate, Dr. Roberts procured an assistant professorship at Kent State University. He remained at Kent State until 1973, rising to the level of associate professor, before returning to the University of Illinois at Urbana-Champaign as an assistant research professor in the Children's Research Center. Glyn Roberts is currently a full professor within the Department of Kinesiology at the University of Illinois.

Professor Roberts has made original research contributions to the sport and exercise psychology field on issues relating to the motivational determinants of achievement and to children's experiences in competitive sport, including research on the use of intervention programs to enhance children's enjoyment of sport. His research work on motivation is undoubtedly his most substantial contribution; four of his papers (Roberts, 1975, 1978; Roberts, Kleiber, & Duda, 1981; Roberts & Pascuzzi, 1979) are among the 32 most cited papers in the recent history of the *Journal of Sport Psychology* (LeUnes et al., 1990). This popularity reflects, of course, not only the impact of Professor Roberts's work but also the dominance of motivation as an area of study within the sport psychology field. Although Roberts's motivation research is clearly concerned with practical issues, it has been strongly theory driven, revolving around the application to the sport context of motivational theories from mainstream psychology (viz., the mechanistic theories of McClelland, 1951, and Atkinson, 1957, and the attributional theory of Weiner, 1972).

Like many of the influential researchers in the human action field, Glyn Roberts has not restricted his contribution to a single research focus or simply to disciplinary issues. He has published work on questions of socialization (e.g., Castine & Roberts, 1974); social facilitation (e.g., Haas & Roberts, 1975); modeling (e.g., Gould & Roberts, 1982); and traditional motor learning and control topics, such as memory (Wallace, DeOreo, & Roberts, 1976). At the professional level, Roberts has contributed to knowledge on the international development of sport psychology (e.g., Roberts, 1973; Roberts & Kimiecik, 1989) as well as to the debates on graduate education within the broader context of the human action field (e.g., Roberts, 1985, 1991). His professional involvement in sport psychology has included terms as the president of NASPSPA and as a member of the managing council of the International Society of Sport Psychology; he has edited *The Sport Psychologist* and served on the editorial boards of the *Journal of Sport Psychology, The International Journal of Sport Psychology*, and the *Research Quarterly*. Professor Roberts has been honored with membership of AAHPERD's Academy of Physical Education.

In this chapter, Glyn Roberts describes the development of his experimentation on motivation and the transitions in theoretical focus his work has taken. Note, in reading his chapter, the role serendipity played in his change in research orientation and the resistance he experienced from his colleagues when he made the paradigm shift from a mechanistic to a cognitive approach to motivation. Compare and contrast Roberts's commitment to the sophistication of cognitive models as a basis for improving our understanding of human performance with the approach advocated by Kelso (chapter 3) for the use of more fundamental sciences (such as physics) as a means of advancing our explanation of human action. Pay particular attention to the crucial distinction Glyn Roberts draws between knowing how to do research and knowing how to ask the right questions. The former is easier to acquire through formal methods of instruction, but the latter is more important for the long-term developments of the field and seems to be a somewhat unique characteristic of influential scientists. In chapter 14 we look at some of the preconditions that appear necessary for asking the right questions in science.

AUTOBIOGRAPHY

As a director of research of graduate students at a major research university, I worry a great deal about the most effective way to both train and educate students to the mysteries and mores of the research enterprise. How does one train a student to be a good scientist when being a good scientist is more than knowing how to collect clean data and to analyze the data appropriately? I find it relatively easy to train students how to do research. At the University of Illinois, we are very fortunate in that we have excellent faculty and courses in research methods and statistics. The excellence of methodologists such as McGrath in psychology and of frontline applied statisticians, as well as our own excellent faculty in the department, enables us to enhance the research skills of students. We simply direct them to the appropriate courses.

Knowing how to do research, however, is not sufficient. One must also know the important questions to ask. This is the most difficult aspect of graduate education: How does one recognize major conceptual steps forward versus interesting, but trivial, side steps? How does one educate students to ask the right questions in their areas of expertise? How does anyone know how to ask the right questions?

Discovery in science is not made through the development of methodology or the use of statistics. Although these are important tools, they only help us to answer the question. The act of discovery comes from the scientist's interpreting the data and deciphering the meaning of the data for the psychological process under investigation. This understanding and insight into the data gives us the steps forward into our understanding of the phenomena pertinent to sport. In sport psychology, I argue, knowledge of concepts and a rethinking of theory have paved our way to understanding. And it is this reconceptualization that has been at the center of advancement in our field, and at the center of advancement of my own research area in motivation. My purpose in this chapter is to attempt to illustrate some of the steps that occur in our understanding of motivation in sport. Our understanding has come about from a rethinking of the meaning of data. Inevitably, I am going to "put my sickle to other people's corn," in that all of us, in our quest to understand psychological phenomena, stand on the shoulders of those who have gone before. But in so doing, I hope to illustrate an important aspect of discovery—the use of theoretical concepts and their application to the issue of understanding motivation in sport. My recollection is personal, and I shall reflect upon my own modest contribution to the advancement of our understanding.

Early Motivation Research

As with most people, my first major piece of research was my doctoral dissertation (Roberts, 1969). I immersed myself in motivation from a conceptual perspective and became engrossed in the measurement technology. When I first began to investigate the issue of motivation in 1967, three conceptual paradigms existed. The first, and the most popular, was the achievement motivation approach of McClelland (1951) and Atkinson (1964); the second was the test anxiety approach of Sarason, Hill, and Zimbardo (1964); and the third was the expectancy of reinforcement approach of Crandall (1963) (see Roberts, 1982). The McClelland-Atkinson approach made the most sense to me at the time, and I followed this approach in my early work.

The McClelland-Atkinson research paradigm is an exemplary model of psychological theorizing and empirical research conducted to verify the constructs. McClelland and associates believed that achievement motives are socialized into the human organism at an early age, thereby becoming an integral part of the organism. Achievement motivation theory states that individuals have one of two motives: the motive to achieve success and the motive to avoid failure. Individuals who are motivated to achieve success choose tasks of intermediate difficulty and try harder and persist longer than individuals who are motivated to avoid failure. In my doctoral dissertation, I used a motor task and investigated risk taking and performance. I predicted both risk-taking and performance differences consistent with the motives.

My research supported the risk-taking hypothesis in that achieve-success individuals preferred intermediate challenge, and avoid-failure individuals avoided intermediate challenge. However, the performance hypotheses were not supported. Achieve-success people did not systematically outperform avoid-failure people (Roberts, 1971). Following my dissertation research, I did several subsequent studies using the same basic paradigm in order to investigate the performance predictions of achievement motivation theory. In none of this research did I systematically support performance hypotheses. This made me very suspicious of the whole approach. In addition, there was a serendipitous finding in my dissertation research that made me question the predictions concerning avoid-failure and achieve-success individuals even more. When I began the project, I asked subjects to come to the testing site twice. The first time subjects performed, I determined the probabilities of success at the task, and they came back on a future occasion to either compete or cooperate on the task. I found that in the first testing period, the achieve-success individuals turned up at the testing site consistently. They were very reliable subjects. But I had a great deal of difficulty persuading the avoid-failure people to come to the testing site. However, late in the semester, when it came time for the subjects to do the task itself in a competitive or cooperative climate, I found the opposite: The achieve-success people frequently would not turn up, whereas the avoid-failure people always turned up. This was an odd reversal of behavior. The only rationale for this was that because the second testing time was during final examinations, the achieve-success people did not come to the experimental site because they considered it more important to work for examinations. Avoid-failure people, on the other hand, readily came to the testing site, because this enabled them to avoid the primary task of working for examinations; this protected the subjects from failure should it occur. This led me to consider, for the first time, the environmental setting in which we were conducting research in motivation and the impact the situation had upon achievement behavior.

I began to question the whole paradigm, because several other aspects bothered me. The paradigm made assumptions that just were not true. It had an ethnocentric bias. Ethnic minorities would often score low on achieve-success measures yet would be highly motivated in some settings such as sport. Further, the paradigm did not describe the achievement of women well and placed too much emphasis upon personality as the crucial variable (see Roberts, 1982). Although the paradigm had a strong conceptual underpinning, the data that we collected just did not ring true consistently in sport. Therefore, I began to consider other conceptual models in which to conduct achievement motivation research.

The Cognitive Approach of Attribution Theory

In 1973, I became aware of a whole new conceptual approach to motivation. I read a book by Weiner et al. (1971) that was one of the first to articulate a cognitive approach to motivation. It became clear that the only acceptable alternative to a mechanistic approach was a cognitive approach to motivation. The cognitive approach to motivation conceives of humans as active information-processing organisms and includes higher mental processes as determinants of action. The approach assumes that individuals seek out information in order to construct a cognitive representation of the environment and that this representation mediates the behavioral response. The essential assumption is that thought precedes action (Roberts, 1984).

Attribution theory deals with the rules individuals use in attempting to account for the causes of behavior. It is a phenomenological approach and attempts to determine the causes of everyday events. To reach causal inference, an individual must search for information, assemble it, and process it. The theory assumes that the causal cognitions mediate between the stimulus and the response through their effect upon affect and expectancy. The important cognitions, which account for achievement behavior, are ability, effort, luck, and task difficulty. These are placed into a framework that includes the dimensions of locus of causality and locus of stability. The attraction of the attribution model was that it overcame many of the criticisms of the Atkinsonian approach (see Roberts, 1982).

I conducted several studies in children's sport programs investigating the causal attributions of children in reaction to winning and losing (e.g., Roberts, 1975). Attribution theory gave significantly more insight into the process of motivation. Whereas the mechanistic model of Atkinson was concerned with individuals who display either high or low achievement motives, attribution theory gave insight into the reasons why individuals are motivated. In particular, the dimensional analysis of Weiner et al. (1971) allowed us to investigate the determinants of motivation, whether our study was centered in the classroom or on the playing field (see Roberts, 1978). The approach was ecologically valid in that it captured the process individuals go through when engaged in sport activities.

As an aside, an interesting phenomenon occurred at about this time. As one of the first people to begin research in attribution theory in sport, I received a great deal of criticism; other motivation researchers resisted the approach. My colleagues argued that the attribution model was much too simplistic and that asking individuals to state how much ability, effort, luck, or task difficulty contributed to outcomes was not even good research. Some of my colleagues argued that asking subjects to respond to questions concerning relative contributions of the attributes was too naive a measurement technology to produce data to meaningfully understand psychological processes. In fact, one senior colleague in 1975 discussed attribution theory as a mere fad and said that the "brushfire" would rapidly burn out. As a relatively young researcher, I really had to defend my position constantly. For me, it was a classic case in which individuals assumed that if the measurement technology was not precise and sophisticated, then it could not be good science. But, as I have stated elsewhere (Roberts, 1989), if a question is not worth asking, it is not worth answering well! In the beginning, attribution research methodology was somewhat basic, but what some people ignored was the profound conceptual issue under discussion. It wasn't until 1978 and later that research work using attribution theory was accepted as being mainstream (albeit with new and improved measurement devices!).

Even though attribution research continues to be an active area, the approach itself has limitations that were beginning to become evident in 1978. The first troubling finding was that causal attributions are not always rational! Attributions have motivational bases in that sometimes people adopt self-serving attributional strategies—variously called self-enhancement, ego-defensive, ego-enhancing, or ego-biased strategies—because individuals are strongly motivated to view themselves in a positive light. Consequently, individuals attribute success and failure to factors that promote the most positive self-image (Roberts, 1978). Although this finding made intuitive sense, it did raise some serious questions relative to the attributions that I asked in my research and to their stability (Brawley & Roberts, 1984).

I began to question whether the attributions of ability, effort, task difficulty, and luck are indeed the major attributions that people use in real settings and whether these remain stable across settings, especially sport. We, as experimenters, had given the subjects the scales, and the players determined how much the attribute contributed to the outcome. We assumed that these elements were the only important causes of sport outcomes. However, I began to argue that the attributes assigned to individuals in sport contexts were not necessarily the same attributes they would use if they responded freely. Therefore, I began to conduct research asking individuals to respond to stimuli qualitatively and to state the causes of presented outcomes.

The important finding (Roberts & Pascuzzi, 1979) was that when allowed to respond freely, subjects identified 11 causal elements. The four traditional elements given to athletes only accounted for 45% of attributions. This was inconsistent with work in the classroom, where 80% of all reported attributions were the traditional four (Frieze, 1976). Further, some attributions, especially ability, were not always viewed as being stable. This meant that the context of sport was different than the context of the classroom. And even though I argued that the attributions used by studies were still pertinent to attribution theory, I began to question the approach of Weiner. What sealed its fate for me was the fact that attribution theory did not help when we wished to suggest means to enhance motivation. Both attribution theory and learned helplessness research (Dweck, 1980) advocate effort attribution retraining to enhance motivation. But in sport, the dominant attribute is ability, not effort, and any motivation enhancement strategy must involve ability attribution retraining (Roberts & Pascuzzi, 1979).

As applied to motivation enhancement, the attributional approach has a fundamental weakness that limits its usefulness in applied settings. Although it provides an excellent conceptual model for a microanalysis of the motivation process and continues to give powerful insights into motivation and achievement behavior, the approach does not provide the conceptual tools educators need to intervene and correct misattributions of performance-debilitating cognitions, such as low ability. The attribution approach is more a paradigm for investigating the social psychology of motivation perception than it is a paradigm for investigating the psychology of motivation (Roberts, 1982). Consequently, its usefulness to sport motivation is limited if we wish to develop intervention strategies to enhance motivation. It became clear, therefore, that the attribution approach has limitations that made many of us working in motivation at the time question its use.

The Cognition Approach of Achievement Goals

The search was on for a better conceptual model and one that incorporated ability attributions. We needed to make better sense of the data we were collecting, especially in terms of motivation enhancement. The learned helplessness model was intuitively appealing (Dweck, 1980) but just did not fit the sport context because it did not involve ability attributions systematically.

A study that convinced me was one that I did with Kevin Spink (Spink & Roberts, 1980). It had always bothered me that winning and losing had been the success and failure criteria by which investigators had applied causal attribution scales to players. It was assumed that winning was success and losing was failure. But success and failure are not synonymous with winning and losing. Indeed, success and failure are better seen as psychological states based upon the individual's interpretation of outcomes. Thus, similar outcomes may elicit different subjective reactions on the part of athletes.

Spink and Roberts (1980) argued that the interpretation of success and failure depends upon whether the individual believes he or she has demonstrated a desirable personal characteristic. Playing against a superior opponent and almost winning is certainly evidence of great effort and ability, both desirable qualities. Objectively, the outcome is still a loss, but it may be interpreted as a success. Thus, the losing player may be satisfied with the performance and perceive the experience as a success. Similarly, a player may be dissatisfied with his or her performance even though the outcome is a victory. Clearly, understanding the individual's interpretation of the outcome is important if we are to understand attributions and cognitions.

To study this, we (Spink & Roberts, 1980) looked at the level of player performance satisfaction following a win or a loss. We identified four categories of players—satisfied winners, dissatisfied winners, satisfied losers, and dissatisfied losers. We asked the subjects to rate their own levels of ability and the levels of ability of their opponents. These ability data were crucial to understanding the perceptions of success and failure and to understanding the cognitions of the players. The data revealed that satisfied winners were those who played against and had beaten competent opponents. Dissatisfied winners believed that they had beaten inferior opponents and attributed their wins to the opponents' lack of ability. Losers had similar perceptions, in that losers beaten by competent opponents felt satisfied with their own performances even though they lost. They felt that they lost because their opponents were just that much better. Losers who lost to mediocre opponents, on the other hand, were very dissatisfied and considered the experience a complete failure. Clearly, although outcomes are sometimes synonymous with success and failure, they are not necessarily so.

When individuals are in sport achievement situations of importance, they are able to accurately assess their own and their opponents' relative abilities. These individuals process information in a logical manner in order to arrive at the cognitions governing performance. Thus, to understand the motivation of an individual, a researcher must understand the perceptions of ability of the individual and understand the ability of the opponent. Clearly, we must take into consideration the complex interpretations athletes make when they define success and failure. The perception of ability and the meaning of achievement to the athletes are crucial to motivation. This is where I began to use the work of Maehr and Nicholls (e.g., 1980) on achievement goals.

As an aside, this was the point at which happenstance affected my thinking, as often happens in science. Maehr, Nicholls, Ames, Dweck, and I were all at the University of Illinois at this time, and we held weekly seminars to discuss our own research agendas. Nicholls was the intellectual leader, and all of us who attended changed our research directions. Long dissatisfied with mechanistic approaches, Maehr and Nicholls (1980) urged that we redefine motivation and rethink the nature of achievement behavior. In order to fully understand achievement motivation and behavior in all its forms, we should take into account the function and meaning of behavior to the individual and should identify the goals of action. It is necessary to understand the subjective meaning of achievement for an individual before we can truly understand achievement behavior.

The first step to understanding achievement behavior is to examine perceptions of success and failure for each individual. Maehr and Nicholls (1980) proposed that three forms of goal orientation existed and that these determined the form of achievement behavior and the criteria of success and failure. These goals are performance-oriented goals, mastery-oriented goals, and social-approval-oriented goals. These are explained elsewhere in detail (Roberts, 1982). These goals have emerged consistently across studies in sport, and one can argue that they are the most relevant to sport and exercise. But two goals in particular have dominated our thinking.

Specifically, the achievement goal approach assumes that the primary focus of individuals in sport achievement context is to demonstrate ability (Nicholls, 1984). But, ability has two concepts in achievement contexts, and these two concepts of ability lead to the development of two goal perspectives in sport. The first goal is performance related—individuals wish to demonstrate higher ability than others (Ames, 1984; Nicholls,

1984). This goal drives achievement behavior in circumstances in which social comparison is the important criterion of comparison. Perceptions of one's own competence are normative and are clearly referenced to the ability of other competitors. Success, or failure, depends upon the subjective assessment of comparing one's own ability with that of relevant others. This goal is termed *ego involvement* by Nicholls (1984), but others call it *performance goal* (Dweck, 1986) or *ability-focused goal* (Ames, 1984). I believe the term *competitive goal* is more pertinent to the context of sport. There is now considerable data to support the existence and relevance of this goal in sport (e.g., Duda, 1992; Roberts, 1992).

The second achievement goal is the goal of demonstrating mastery or learning of the activity in sport (Nicholls, 1984). This goal drives achievement behavior in circumstances in which learning or mastering the task is deemed important. Competence is self-referenced and dependent upon learning. Success, or failure, depends on the subjective assessment of whether one has improved or learned on a task. This goal is termed *task involvement* by Nicholls (1984), but others call it *learning goal* (Dweck, 1986), or *mastery goal* (Ames, 1984). In sport, I prefer the term mastery goal. Again, considerable data support the existence and relevance of this goal in sport (e.g., Duda, 1992; Roberts, 1992).

Multiple goals exist and do interact with the sporting situation in meaningful ways. For example, Ewing (1981) studied the question directly and found that achievement goals do exist in sport and that these achievement goals do affect achievement behavior. The major finding of Ewing was that dropping out of sport is related to a competitive goal orientation.

Clearly, to understand the achievement behavior of athletes, we need to understand their goal orientation toward the demonstration of ability. The work of Duda (1989), among others, has confirmed that a very important element in sport motivation is the goal orientation of the athlete.

The essential aspect of Nicholls's work (1984, 1989) is its consistency with my own perception of the focus of the athlete's attention within the sport situation: the individual's perception of his or her capacity in relation to others. In sport, the focus of attention is on the self, and one compares one's performance to the level of effort and performance of others in order to assess one's ability. Therefore, understanding ability assessment is important.

Assessing ability in sport is very complex and involves at least three evaluations. One is an assessment of the ability of the opponent in relation to all other opponents: Is the opponent a weak or a strong player? Second, how does one's own ability compare to the opponent's ability? And third, how much effort is applied by oneself and by the opponent? The assessment of opponent's and one's own competence in sport contexts involves social comparison processes (Roberts, 1984). Because of the social comparison processes involved, the outcome is salient and unambiguous in sport. All participants and observers can readily observe who won and lost.

The importance of the outcome is often exacerbated by the coach. Coaches are very outcome oriented, and coaching folklore is replete with sayings such as "Winning isn't everything, it's the only thing." The pervasive belief seems to be that it is not how you play the game, it is whether you win or lose that is important.

The total effect of this outcome orientation, and the inherent pressure on athletes to use social comparison processes, is to enhance the perception of ability as the most important mediator of achievement and motivation and to force athletes to develop competitive goal orientations. The tragic aspect for those of us in motivation research is the fact that because of the outcome orientation of coaches, children use outcome as the criterion of success and failure. If they lose, they lack ability! In reality, these players may be very able. But children do not use self-referenced criteria in these situations (Roberts, 1984), and this comes out clearly in our interviews with children. Thus, we develop in children, and in athletes in general, the perception that the most important goal orientation to hold is a competitive goal orientation.

This research, and that of others (e.g., Ames, 1992), made me sensitive to the psychological climate created by coaches. The climate we create leads to the development of achievement goals. And in sport, the achievement goal of competitiveness is the most prominent. But the evidence is clear that if we want to help athletes and enhance motivation, we must enhance the development of mastery goals. But how can we do that? This question has concerned me in my research of late. If we need to imbue athletes with mastery cognitions, how can we do this so that we enhance the motivation of athletes (Roberts, 1984)?

A student (Burton, 1983) at Illinois set up a goal-setting program that focused upon enhancing mastery cognitions. The investigation tested two general hypotheses. First, does goal setting teach athletes to set appropriate goals? Second, do athletes who set effective goals have cognitions consistent with those of people who are mastery oriented? Burton's results supported the first hypothesis; the swimmers who set goals focused on performance goals that made them more realistic in their performance expectancies. Of importance in this context, the second hypothesis was supported in that swimmers who set goals demonstrated significantly more mastery cognitions than those who did not. Another student (Hall, 1990) also investigated the goal-setting phenomenon in terms of creating a mastery climate and confirmed that motivation in physical contexts is better served when we create mastery climates. Further, research I have currently underway demonstrates that to enhance motivation of children in extracurricular activities, we should create mastery motivational climates in sport. In other words, creating mastery climates enhances the mastery goal orientation and encourages athletes to persist.

There is an obvious need for more research in this area, but the research must be directed at understanding why motivation ebbs and flows within the sport context. This is why I think all of us in motivational research need to understand the conceptual underpinning to motivation, so that when we apply our intervention strategies, these strategies emanate from an understanding of the determinants of achievement behavior. Even though I still argue for a convergence of existing approaches to help us better understand the process of motivation in sport (Roberts, 1992), I must agree with Nicholls (1992), who argues that we will advance our understanding of motivation in sport if we focus more on the specific social cognitive dynamics of the sport environment and how these affect achievement behaviors.

Future Directions in Motivation Research

We must continue to move ahead on the conceptual front. Great strides are being made. The variables I have mentioned thus far (motivational climate, achievement goal, and perception of ability) are critical variables in any model to understand motivation. Such models must incorporate the multivariate complexity of the sport situation, because such models are more likely to capture the individual and social realities of people in sport. We must move away from the simplistic linear processing models. In the real world, effects are the result of multiple causes in complex interaction. In sport motivation, we must spend more time creating hypotheses that emanate from an understanding of the social dynamics of the individual in sport. We need to describe, document, and represent the social cognitive functioning of the sport participant. Only then can we begin to consider the appropriate intervention strategies that may amend particular cognitive deficits undergirding deviant, inappropriate, or ineffectual behavior (Roberts, 1989).

Sport psychologists should spend more time considering hypothesis generation and less time worrying about how to collect and analyze data. Both tasks are essential to the research enterprise, but the creative phase is clearly the most important. If our questions are inappropriate, or trivial, then why bother collecting data in the first place (Roberts, 1989)?

The insights into motivation in sport thus far have come from a conceptual understanding of the variables that matter. It is not appropriate to blindly follow models from psychology. Rather, we have utilized these models and observed their fit into the sport setting. And, it is this fitting of the dirty data of the real sporting world into a conceptual framework that has advanced our understanding of motivation and will continue to do so in the future.

Chapter 13

Brent S. Rushall

Department of Physical Education
College of Professional Studies and Fine Arts
San Diego State University
San Diego, California, U.S.A.

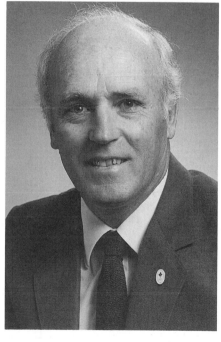

Born in Sydney, Australia, in 1939, and educated at Sydney Boys' High School, Brent Rushall completed a diploma in physical education (with honors) from Sydney Teachers' College in 1960. He continued part-time study toward a BA from the University of Sydney from 1961 to 1964 while holding full-time teaching appointments (first at Sydney Boys' High School and later at Sefton High School) as well as a part-time swim coaching position at Forbes Carlile's School of Swimming. Rushall moved to the United States in 1965, completing a master's degree in exercise physiology in 1967 and a PhD in human performance in 1969 under the supervision, in both cases, of Dr. James "Doc" Counsilman at Indiana University. After returning to Sydney for 2 years and working as a systems engineer for IBM Australia, he moved to Halifax, Canada, in 1971 to a teaching and research position in the School of Physical Education at Dalhousie University. After 4 years at Dalhousie and a further 10 in the School of Physical Education and Outdoor Recreation at Lakehead

University, Dr. Rushall moved back to the United States in 1985 to his current position as professor within the Department of Physical Education at San Diego State University.

Brent Rushall has made a unique contribution to the sport and exercise psychology field and to the sports coaching sphere through his adoption of the behavioristic, operant-conditioning methods of B.F. Skinner to the problems of human performance enhancement in exercise and sport. He has written extensively on the behavior patterns of elite athletes and especially on the application of behavioral analysis and modification schedules to applied problems in sport (e.g., Rushall, 1975b, 1978a, 1980; Rushall & Fry, 1980; Rushall & Leet, 1979; Rushall & Smith, 1979); this work has been extremely influential at the coach and athlete level. Professor Rushall has, throughout his career, been an outspoken critic of the predominant use of cognitive models by other sport and exercise psychology theorists and experimenters, noting that the arbitrary nature of the mechanisms proposed within cognitive models makes them untestable within the normal methods of natural science. The tests of behaviorism Professor Rushall outlines in his chapter necessitate a research interest in real-world problems and a paradigmatic preference for single-subject research designs of a type that is unusual in the majority of human action research. For this reason, it is not surprising that Rushall has made his greatest impact in the applied sphere and has willingly involved himself as a consultant to many international-caliber sports performers. For example, he has been sport psychologist to Canadian Olympic teams in swimming, wrestling, ski jumping, and cross-country skiing; has held coaching appointments in swimming, rugby, and rowing; and has launched an international firm for sport psychology consultation. This activity has provided Professor Rushall with the basis for a dynamic interaction between theory and practice. Rushall has served on the editorial boards of the *Canadian Journal of Applied Sport Sciences*, the *Journal of Sport Psychology*, and the *Journal of Applied Research in Coaching and Athletics*, and he has been honored professionally with fellowship to the International Society of Sport Psychology.

In reading Brent Rushall's autobiography of his experiences in sport and exercise psychology experimentation, focus on the stark contrast in theoretical orientation between his work and that of Carron, Nideffer, and especially Roberts. Note, despite significant differences in Rushall's and Kelso's theoretical positions, the parallels between the criticisms Rushall levels at the cognitive approach to sport and exercise psychology and the criticisms Kelso levels at the cognitive approach to motor learning and control. Observe how Rushall's own preference for a behavioristic approach was molded in part by his real-world educational experiences as a computer engineer, and share in the frustration he has experienced with behavioral theory's failure to attain paradigmatic dominance in the sport and exercise psychology field, despite its apparent effectiveness as a practical means of enhancing human performance. Also, note the range of teachers and high-level coaches and athletes who have helped shape Brent Rushall's career and the chance events that shifted his orientation from physiologist to psychologist.

AUTOBIOGRAPHY

During my school days in Sydney, Australia, I aspired to great heights in sporting performance. With a limited physical capacity, I did not achieve those aspirations to my satisfaction. I had been greatly influenced by my rowing coaches at Sydney Boys' High School, the late Frank Nicolls, and the late Alan Callaway, who went on to coach the Australian silver-medal eight at the Mexico Olympic Games. While still a college student in the late 1950s, I was thrust into coaching Olympic athletes despite a lack of experience. This seemed to be an adventitious diversion for my aspirations. I had started to work as an assistant to the world-renowned coach-scientist Forbes Carlile. My studies in physical education were very enjoyable and it was in them that my academic curiosity was aroused. These setting events, and their associated contingencies, initiated my desire to discover how to control the performances of top-class athletes.

My initial studies were in exercise physiology (Rushall, 1960, 1967c). While teaching and coaching in the early 1960s, I also took another undergraduate degree at night at Sydney University in the fields of psychology and philosophy. Those were the only course options that were available for my schedule at that time.

During the late 1950s and first half of the 1960s, I continued to train athletes in a physiological sense but was somewhat frustrated by my inability to control their development in any consistent fashion. It appeared that physiological training alone was not the complete answer for helping athletes develop their fullest potentials. Although my psychological training at that time was Freudian, with a strong emphasis on measurement and evaluation, courses I completed contained odd snippets of information that suggested ways to control subjects, whether they be animal or human. I attempted to communicate those features (Rushall, 1965).

After the Tokyo Olympic Games, I went to Indiana University to complete a master's degree. This was to be a stopover during my world travels, which were the wont of Australian youth at that time. James "Doc" Counsilman was my adviser and good friend while I was at IU. He encouraged my studies in psychology because he viewed that as the new frontier for sports improvement. The academic license and course excellence that existed at IU allowed me to pursue a course of studies that best suited my interests. Although my master's degree was in exercise physiology, and the impact of the late Sid Robinson on my life-long interest in physiology cannot be understated, I exploited all the opportunities to study and get involved in psychology, philosophy of science, and measurement. Doc Counsilman directed both of my degree theses, and I was fortunate enough to be the first PhD graduate in human performance (double major in psychology and evaluation) from IU. The association with Doc and his great swimmers of that era and the involvement with John Pont's Rose Bowl football team and Lou Watson's champion basketball team kept me attuned to the need to consider all aspects of an athlete in the quest for sporting excellence.

At IU I was greatly influenced by the late Frank Restle in understanding the paramount role of learning in the development of human behavior, by Irving Saltzman for understanding the potential and tenets of operant psychology, and by Nick Fattu for developing an appreciation of good evaluation and measurement. Art Slater-Hammel instilled a desire for rigor that has stayed with me to this day. Those great academic teachers, along with the applied concerns and quests of Forbes and Doc, inspired me to embrace operant psychology (which was then referred to as *behavior modification*) as the psychological bent that would best serve the practitioner (Rushall, 1967a, 1967b, 1970b).

Upon returning to Australia in the middle of 1969, I worked for IBM Australia Limited, becoming a systems engineer after completing the company's intensive education programs. I found that the theoretical courses that I had studied were of little use in the real world, whereas the principles of behavior modification were extremely helpful to me in designing human-machine systems in the world of computers. The concentration of reinforcing experiences that I had in the business world solidified my belief that operant psychology was the primary psychological focus for practitioners (Rushall, 1978a). At about the same time Daryl Siedentop and I wrote the book *The Development and Control of Behavior in Sport and Physical Education* (Rushall & Siedentop, 1972). This focusing led me to an avowed disdain of the trait approach to understanding behavior (Rushall, 1970a, 1971, 1975c, 1978a) and to development of the description of the philosophical bases for studying applied sport psychology (Rushall, 1978a).

Until recently, the applied behavior analysis approach for studying sport has not been widely accepted. However, it seems that opinions are changing as Daryl, his students, my former students, and I continue to spread the word. It has always been frustrating to gain acceptance outside of one's field before gaining acceptance from within. This has been particularly true with measurement. The formation of behavior analysis inventories (Rushall, 1975b, 1978b, 1985b) as a means for practitioners to understand the behaviors of athletes has received little attention from applied sport psychologists, although behavior therapists have accepted it as a valuable and viable process for measuring behavior (Franks, 1979). The propensity for sport psychologists to want to develop and use tools that produce scale scores is alarming. I have never been able to understand why a scientist would want to discard information, as occurs when a researcher removes response behaviors to a questionnaire when forming a scale score. That approach never did appeal to me (Rushall, 1974, 1978a).

With regard to understanding and demonstrating control over behavior, applied behavior analysis indicates a number of single-subject and small-group designs for investigating questions concerning human behavior. Reversal designs (McKenzie & Rushall, 1974; Rushall & MacEachern, 1977), multiple-baseline designs (Rushall & Smith, 1979), changing criterion designs (Rushall, 1975a), and most recently alternating treatment designs (Chorkawy, 1982; Ford, 1982; McKinnon, 1985; Rushall, 1985a) have provided the answers that often frustrate researchers trying to use traditional intergroup/statistical research designs. Having used both approaches to experimental research, I still am amazed at how much more one understands about the process and progress of an experiment when using single-subject designs as opposed to traditional group studies. Single-subject research is so much more rewarding for the researcher.

The advocacy of applied behavior analysis as the research orientation for applied sport psychology requires the exposition of basic tenets for research. To understand this advocacy, I will discuss some of the major points made in my 1978a paper.

Unacceptable Postulates

To produce a scientific study of both covert and overt behavior, one must have an adequate and satisfactory system of postulates. Kantor (1966) enumerated four untenable research approaches of psychologists that deny them the acceptability of being called scientists. Those approaches are described briefly here.

* *The phenomenological position.* The assumption of "internal" processes, such as experience and states of consciousness, deviates from the scientific rule of confining studies to some definite class of events that are objectively verifiable. Among other things, the data of phenomenological concepts are inaccessible to scientific handling (Lichtenstein, 1971). The assumption that behavior is caused by some occult determining factor, not derived from any contact with events, is not the stuff of science.

* *Mind-body postulates.* The dualistic notion that there exist both a mind and a body maintains an insoluble mystery in science. The crucial fault of this dualism is the lack of explanation of the bridging mechanism between the physical and mental. Adherents assert that at some point the two are linked. The argument to the contrary, that physical and mental

events are compatible, that is, they are behaviors, is persuasive (Pole, 1958). Science requires proof to substantiate entities. The inadequacies of the dualistic notion do not provide the complete proof that produces scientific acceptance. A psychologist should be aware of attempts to offer causal explanations based on the dualistic postulate.

• *Psychic expressions and manifestations.* That mental states are experienced and manifested in behavior is clearly a subtheme of the mind-body postulate. However, feelings and emotional behaviors are unique types of behavior in special kinds of circumstances and can be investigated with a natural science strategy (Kantor, 1966; Lichtenstein, 1971).

• *The organocentric postulate.* This implies that the behavior of individuals is energized by some internal force often called a stimulus or cue. That is, the origin of behavior emanates from within the organism. Historically, the energizer was believed to be the soul, which led to concepts of free will and other such notions. Such a position is insufficient because it contains a logical fallacy—it tries to describe or explain a complicated series of factors in terms of a single or very few factors.

These four postulates are rejected because they do not allow one to embrace a natural science form of inquiry.

Acceptable Postulates

The metapostulates of scientific inquiry that regulate the operations of investigation are applicable to psychology and are as follows:

• *The homogeneity axiom.* The nature and availability of data and events are similar for all scientific fields. Thus, psychologists must be concerned with natural and confrontable events.

• *The independence axiom.* Each science is concerned with an event field. One cannot borrow the abstractions from other sciences and regard them as original data. In the field of physical activity study, this violation is evidenced by the attempt to use communication theory as an analogized explanatory model for motor performance.

• *The nonreduction postulate.* The events studied should be retained. When lawful (functional) relationships are obtained using original events, their further reduction is nonsensical. The belief that reducing behaviors to inferred entities and biological structures produces better experimentation and findings is wrong.

• *The axiom of construct derivation.* No descriptions can be imposed on the original events of an investigation. This denies the introduction of extraneous variables or inferred structures into explanatory and descriptive situations.

Six further axioms indicate the bounds of inquiry for psychology to remain as a form of natural science. The first four concern the data of psychology; the final two embrace the scope of inquiry.

• *Psychological events consist of multifactor interbehavioral fields.* Individuals interact with environmental circumstances in measurable and observable forms.

• *Interbehavioral fields are integral and coordinate.* All factors in a specific behavior segment are of equal importance. It is not acceptable to consider one aspect of the total field, such as an individual's behavior, to be more important than another.

• *Interbehavioral fields are symmetrical and reciprocal.* Behaviors and stimuli occur simultaneously and not as a series of discrete events. An individual behaves as an adjustment to environmental situations. Behavior is not aroused by some preceding event that is removed before the act is evidenced.

• *Interbehavioral fields are evolutional.* Patterns and occurrences of behavior are determined by an individual's history of interactions with the environment. Few exceptions to this axiom exist (e.g., respondent behaviors).

• *Interbehavioral fields are outgrowths of ecological behavior.* Psychological behaviors are influenced by the phylogenetic continuum. They are derivations and elaborations of biological activities and are adjustments as part of an evolutionary pattern.

• *Psychological fields permit investigative analysis.* Interbehavioral fields are open to specific study projects. However, this does not allow one to construct the notion that the field consists of parts. Arbitrary, focused investigations should not attach special significance to indicators within the total field. Events must be interpreted in perspective to the entire behavior field.

These postulates allow one to investigate covert and overt behaviors as events that are within the realm of natural science. The main hurdle for the observation of some of these events is the technologies available. Consequently, the statures of these tenets often have been violated for ease and expediency of producing pseudoscientific work that is often contingent upon powerful reinforcement.

There are a number of misconceptions about applied behavior analysts and their work. At one time or another, these misconceptions have been leveled at me, but I have refrained from being overly aversive in my responses. The remainder of this paper will discuss some of the misunderstandings (Day, 1969).

Facts comprise measurable and observable indicators. Skinner (1950) advocated a rejection of "any explanation of an observed fact which appeals to events taking place somewhere else at some other level of observation, described in different terms, and measured, if at all, in different dimensions" (p. 193). This amounts to a rejection of terminologies that imply purpose, drives, and fanciful states such as aggression, creativity, and anxiety. This process of abstraction constructs a world that is never directly experienced. Philosophically, this process is unsound because it is substantiated by circular argument: Abstractions are defined in terms of facts they are supposed to explain. The absurdity of this latter point is illustrated in the following dialogue for the concept of anxiety.

1. A set of behaviors is observed.
2. The question is asked, "Why did he do those things?"
3. The answer is provided, "Because he was anxious."
4. The explanation is then questioned, "How do you know he was anxious?"
5. The answer is provided, "Because he did those things."

This process of substantiation exists for all constructs (explanatory fictions or panchrestons). Until a person's anxiousness can be manipulated as an independent variable it cannot be objectively verified to exist. When the day arrives that the subject can be made to behave at 50% of anxiety level and then altered to function at 75% of anxiety level, I will retract this assertion. Unfortunately, the majority of the behaviors of psychologists involve such fictional constructs, the psychologists being safe in the understanding that the concepts about which they speak can never be disproved or substantiated.

The use of explanatory constructs to account for behavior is not acceptable. Because such constructs are not available for measurement or observation, it becomes necessary for the protagonists of mental constructs to prove the existence of these constructs rather than for the antimentalists to prove nonexistence of the constructs. However, neither proof nor disproof can be accomplished satisfactorily.

In the history of behaviorism, overt and covert behaviors were originally considered. However, the more problematical covert behaviors were neglected, which led to the impression that they were denied as behaviors. Such a denial is not acceptable. The measurement and analysis of covert behavior is possible within a single framework. However, the measurement of covert behaviors (thinking behaviors) is usually beyond the reach of science. The current advances in technology are bringing covert behaviors closer to observation and measurement, so that the future holds promise for exciting new investigations. Generally, though, one can only infer private events from behaviors; that is, a verbal report is a behavioral response to private events. That interpretation contrasts markedly with the common belief that a verbal report is a sensation. Within sport psychology research, researchers still attempt to influence thinking behaviors at a level external to the individual. My current projects involve manipulating external instructions and stimuli that suggest different types of thinking (Crossman, 1977; Rushall, 1975d, 1979, 1982, 1984, 1986, 1992; Selkirk, 1980; Shewchuk, 1985). That research does not advocate that thoughts are changed; it only assesses the functional relationship between certain setting events and behaviors.

We should also contemplate another consideration of the internal events that occur in humans. Language is learned and is a reaction to responses to physical events from internal and external environments. If it is not, then how can there be so many different languages and dialects? The learning process entails differential reinforcement. Many schools of psychology and philosophy exist today because of differential reinforcement contingencies associated with the learning of language rather than because of some consistent well-founded philosophy of science. Thus, contingencies in a psychologist's life determine whether he or she embraces subjectivity or objectivity in the scientific approach to psychology. Unfortunately, the contingencies that support subjectivity and verbal avoidance behaviors are very much in force today.

That so much unscientific work exists in sport psychology can be explained by the construction of language. We can determine reasons for verbalizing and reasons for the content of verbalizations through the analysis of contingencies of reinforcement. For example, we learn a repertoire of verbal statements concerning emotions that are appropriate in differentiated situations and lead to reinforcement. Therefore, language is a behavior that is analogous to any other behavior. Labels are proposed in the language to differentiate emotions despite the fact that the underlying physiological states of most emotions are similar. A psychological laboratory that has a number of armchairs as its equipment is not a scientific milieu but rather a rich source of intriguing contingencies governing the use of language. This is an operant interpretation of many of the schools of psychology. Scientific conferences are much more interesting if, in most sessions, a listener attempts to discern why a speaker projects the content of a talk rather than if the listener takes the content of the talk seriously. That fact will reveal much more about behavior than will the consideration of most presented topics.

There are no such things as meanings (mental entities focally involved in communication). Meaning is verbal usage. By adopting such a position we can avoid the translation problem of paraphrasing and the circularity of argument just illustrated. Meaning becomes an understanding of why verbal behaviors occur. The discovery of the conditions under which language is emitted and why each response is controlled by its corresponding conditions produces more meaningful meaning. In this framework, meaning consists of whatever makes us think we know anything.

A final feature of an acceptable psychology for sport is that there should be a focus on description and control rather than explanation. This position opposes being hypothetical or theoretical. According to Skinner (1938), terms "are used merely to bring together groups of observations, to state uniformities, and to express properties of behavior which transcend single instances" (p. 44). Thus, there are no hypotheses to be proved or disproved, but rather there is a need to produce convenient representations of things already known. The regressive asking of *why* is nothing but a language game; it adds nothing to the control of behavior. It is better to be an observer of natural contingencies; that is the province of science. Embracing ontology is of little use.

The considerations I have just outlined have limited and directed my approaches to understanding human behavior, particularly in the realm of sports. One further contemplation will describe a behavioral outcome of the contingencies that have shaped my life. It concerns the methodology of science. Is the hypothetico-deductive (HD) or the positivistic-inductive (PI) method more appropriate? The principal weakness of the PI approach concerns the decision criteria for leaping from particular to universal propositions. The decision criteria concern the characteristics of certainty and representativeness. Their use and influence vary markedly.

Contemporary fashion favors the HD method or constructional dogma of method and theory. The contingencies surrounding adherence to this approach are many. Its use is often substantiated through analogy to the mistaken belief that the physical sciences owe their modern pragmatic success to their constructional theoretical systems. Often HD fictions are proposed as substitutes for facts; that is, they are panchrestons and they flourish where facts (data) are few. In the topical realities of many academic-scientific areas we are familiar with quotations and sayings that recognize this assertion (e.g., certain bovine excrements baffle brains). The criticisms of the HD method are many, but there are two that I should emphasize in this discussion. The first concerns the nature of theorizing. Typically, a theory is originated through a mixture of an individual's fantasy and very limited, adventitious observation. The second embraces the basis of theory. A theory has unchallengeable axioms as beginnings that contain terms that need no definitions. This poses a problem. Where do the axioms initially come from? The resultant purpose of HD research becomes one of proving propositions right or wrong rather than learning something about the world. In many HD studies, important events in life are ignored because they are outside the scope of the investigation. In a very strict sense, assumptions, axioms, predictions, and postulates are guesses. Thus, the postulates of both methods are generated in the same way. A decision as to which method of reasoning is preferred is based upon the conditions that surround a scientist's endeavors. The natural scientist will employ the positivistic-inductive method of inquiry. From a personal viewpoint, I have always learned much more from single-subject experimentation than from intergroup strategies. Those positively reinforcing experiences increase the probability that I will continue in that fashion.

Skinner (1983) recounted three Baconian principles that have characterized his personal life, which (in true followership form) I believe are also appropriate to my own mode of inquiry. Those principles are as follows:

- Study nature, not books. Books must follow sciences, not sciences books.

  I have read for pleasure but less often to learn, and I am poorly read in psychology—that is one of the ways in which I "neglect my contemporaries." My experiments came out of other experiments, not out of theories. My books were written out of nature, not out of other books. (p. 407)

- Nature, to be commanded, must be obeyed.
- A better world will result from planning and building, not from chance happenings.

The events that have shaped my approach to scientific discovery have centered around three sources. The first source is the teachers with whom I have been fortunate to be associated: Frank Restle, Irving Saltzman, Art Slater-Hammel, and Nick Fattu at Indiana University and B.F. Skinner through his many writings and clear communications. The vicarious reinforcement I experienced in their classes and presence remains vivid when compared to all my other learning experiences. The second source is the association between science and high-level sport. Forbes Carlile, Jim Counsilman, Don Talbot, my fellow students at Indiana University, Daryl Siedentop, and Frank Pyke, encouraged that interest and a concern for scientific method and control. The frequency of reinforcement that occurs when applied scientific principles are used in coaching athletes has generated a high rate of behavior in this field for me. The students who have studied with me and with whom I have been fortunate to work also have contributed much to the modification of my own scientific behavior. They have been a rich source of behavior and information, and associating with them in a close manner has yielded much positive reinforcement. The third source is the interactions with elite athletes who since 1959 have been willing to serve as subjects in many of my projects. The gratitude that I owe to Canadian, Australian, and American Olympians, who tolerated measurements and observations in many important competitive settings, is more than I can ever repay. The continued reinforcement that has occurred through associations with these persons has contributed to my persistence in observing events in the sporting world that control and describe behavior. The modification of my own behavior was generated largely by those persons and environments that I have mentioned here.

Part V

Experimentation in Action:
Observations
of Expert Experimenters

W e have examined in Part I the construct of experimentation and the potential impact of the experimenter upon all stages of the experimentation process. We have since seen in Parts II through IV experimentation described from a first-person perspective by noted experimenters in motor learning and control, motor development, and sport and exercise psychology. These autobiographies provide unique insights into the impact of personal and situational factors upon the experimentation process and insight into how experimenters generate research ideas and make critical decisions throughout all parts of the experimentation process. Chapter 14 provides a synthesis of the preceding autobiographical chapters and further comment on a number of the issues and themes presented in chapter 1.

We focus, in particular, on the question of expertise in experimentation, searching for commonalities in approach and in personal characteristics among the expert experimenters assembled here. Identifying the characteristics of expert experimenters in the human action field is important both for understanding more about the experimentation process per se and for extracting some informed guidelines as to how tertiary education in the movement sciences might best be structured in order to foster the development of such expertise (cf. Newell, 1987). In this chapter, the prime database for an assessment of the characteristics of successful experimenters is the autobiographical accounts of research provided in Parts II through IV of this book, although this information is also supplemented by available autobiographical accounts of eminent psychologists (e.g., Cattell, 1984; Cohen, 1977; Krawiec, 1974; Siegal & Zeigler, 1976). The first-person descriptions of the research experience by noted human action experimenters are shown in this chapter to be largely consistent with accounts of expert researchers from other fields of science (e.g., Gleick, 1987; Zuckerman, 1975), with recent theoretical attempts to outline the genesis of scientific genius (e.g., Langley, Simon, Bradshaw, & Zytkow, 1987; Simonton, 1988, 1989), and with some global notions about cognitive expertise (e.g., J.R. Anderson, 1982; Chi, 1981) that suggest that the ability to recognize structural links between previously unrelated fields and concepts is an essential basis for expertise. Chapter 14 first examines the diversity of the experimentation and research decisions that are made by expert experimenters and then focuses more directly upon expertise as the ability to induce paradigm shifts within a given field of study.

Chapter 14

Expertise in Experimentation on Human Action

Bruce Abernethy

One thing that is immediately striking from a superficial inspection of the preceding autobiographical accounts is the diversity of these experimenters as a group. Although they all have made substantial contributions to the understanding of human action through experimentation, they have done so by converging on the problems of the field from many different backgrounds and by using vastly varying theories, methods, and investigative paradigms. There are clearly many pathways to successful experimentation on human action; for this reason, attempting to outline a prescriptive pathway for experimentation in the motor learning and control, motor development, and sport and exercise psychology fields would be both overly constraining and unrepresentative of experimentation as it occurs in practice. In the first part of this chapter, we explore the extent of diversity in the experimenters themselves (their personalities, backgrounds, and interests) and in the type of experimentation they conduct (their selection of levels of analysis, type of experimental setting, and type of statistical/analytical method). In the second part of this chapter, we go beyond the superficial differences between expert experimenters in search of some more fundamental similarities in mode of thinking, research strategy, and organization of knowledge.

Diversity in Human Action Experimenters and Experimentation

It is apparent from chapters 2 through 13 that expert experimenters in the motor learning and control, motor development, and sport and exercise psychology fields display a wide range of individual differences in (a) their educational backgrounds and experiences in other fields, (b) in their orientations toward research, and (c) in their experimentation styles. In this section we examine the extent of this diversity and compare it with that known to exist in other groups of elite scientists.

Where Do the Expert Researchers Come From and How Do They Get Interested in Human Action Research?

This book has noted at a number of points that the closest parent discipline to all three areas of human action research is experimental psychology. A useful starting point for examining how expert experimenters first become exposed to and interested in research in human action is to consider some parallel evidence that already exists from studies of eminent experimental psychologists. The works of Roe (1952a, 1952b) and Cohen (1977) suggest the following to be generally true about the introduction of eminent psychologists to research in the field of psychology.

Many eminent psychologists, unlike biologists and physicists, become involved in their field more by accident than by design. A childhood and school-age interest in psychology is rare for eminent psychologists, whereas a lifelong interest in the subject matter of the field appears to be somewhat of a prerequisite for involvement in research in biology and physics (Roe, 1953). Expert researchers in psychology, while reaching their profession indirectly, are frequently older when they make their impact on the field than are comparable experts in the more traditional science fields. Often expert researchers reach the field of psychology because of the influence of a particular teacher rather than because of any specific, long-standing interest in the subject matter of the field. Yet despite reaching psychology by accident, many eminent psychologists remain profoundly influenced both by their early training (e.g., see Cohen, 1977, pp. 332-333) and by their experiences as graduate students. The impact of influential teachers and supervisors seems to be a particularly powerful one. Not only do promising researchers tend to gravitate toward successful researchers, but also it appears true that success, to a great degree, creates success in scientific research (e.g., Newell, 1987; Zuckerman, 1975).

The important question in the current context is whether expert researchers in human action are attracted to their subject matter for the same reasons, and through the same routes, as eminent researchers from the parent discipline. The first point that is apparent is that although some eminent researchers reach the fields of human action somewhat by accident and at a mature age (e.g., Henry, and to some degree, Whiting; see chapters 2 and 5), for the majority, a research career in human action is simply a natural progression from personal interest in motor skills as a sports performer, a teacher-coach, or both. One can argue that the research interests of Nideffer, Kelso, and Carron, for instance, have taken root in their sport interests as participants in the martial arts, rugby, and American football, respectively, whereas the research interests of Whiting, Rarick, Keogh, and Rushall can be traced to practical involvement in sport tasks at the teacher/coach level.

When one considers the autobiographies in this book in tandem with the author profiles contained in edited texts such as those by Silva and Weinberg (1984), Unestahl (1983), or Kelso (1982a), it is apparent that there is a very high preponderance of active sporting backgrounds among researchers in the human action field. Unlike researchers in mainstream psychology, researchers in the human action fields appear to frequently have considerable life-long interests and affinities for their subject matter. This experiential background may provide many human action researchers with unique personal insights into their subject matter, and this tacit knowledge (as Polanyi, 1958, 1967, argued) may be extremely useful in the formulation of appropriate questions and hypotheses. A surprising number of human action researchers (e.g., Henry, Kelso, Rushall) have also reached their current interest areas via exercise physiology, a point that tends to indicate an initial general interest in the movement sciences rather than any specific links with the methods and theories of psychology.

A second point that is apparent from examination of the backgrounds of expert human action researchers is that as in mainstream psychology, outstanding teachers and researchers often serve as crucial role models and inspirations for beginning researchers in the human action fields. Significant teachers appear to exert extremely pervasive influences upon those who ultimately become expert researchers, thus setting in progress an important "masters and apprentices" cycle (Newell, 1987). Obvious examples within the movement science field are the influences of the three H's, Slater-Hammel, Henry, and Hubbard (Newell, 1987); Carron's tribute (chapter 10) to the influence of Henry is a good case in point. Other examples of outstanding influence within the autobiographical chapters are the influences of McCloy and Tuttle on Rarick (chapter 7), Counsilman on Rushall (chapter 13), and Keogh on Sugden (chapter 8).

Although significant teachers, especially in the role of postgraduate supervisor, are apparent in the backgrounds of many of our eminent human action researchers, such teachers are neither a necessary nor sufficient condition for success as an experimenter. The early career of Singer (chapter 4) provides a good example of graduate work undertaken with minimal direct supervision. Where significant teachers are present they may act both in inciting interest in science and in providing the young experimenters with a role model, especially with respect to work ethics and practices. The presence of an established researcher as a supervisor may be particularly valuable to a young scientist early in his or her career in boosting initial research productivity (what Simonton, 1977 termed "creative precocity") but may in the long term inhibit lifetime productivity (Simonton, 1987), especially if the apprenticeship experience does not expose the young investigator to all the creative elements of research, beginning with idea formation and terminating with the reporting and publication of the collected data.

Of central importance in the development of scientists who ultimately obtain eminence is exposure to diversified, enriched environments both in childhood and in the early days of their research careers (Simonton, 1987) and opportunity for developing scientists to experiment with all facets of the experimentation process. If the formal education process does not provide this stimulation and opportunity for dabbling in individual creativity, it may act against the development of experimental thinking. Einstein, for instance, suggested that

> It is, in fact, nothing short of a miracle that the modern methods of instruction have not yet entirely strangled the holy curiosity of inquiry; for this delicate little plant, aside from stimulation, stands mostly in need of freedom; without this it goes to wreck and ruin without fail. It is a very grave mistake to think that the enjoyment of seeing and searching can be promoted by means of coercion and a sense of duty. (Schlipp, 1951, p. 17)

Nideffer, in chapter 11, reflects similar sentiments about the inadequacies of formal education in motivating him toward a creative career in sport psychology.

Aside from formal education and the influence of superiors and/or significant teachers, a number of other situational factors may impact upon the career development of eminent human action researchers. In particular, family background appears to have a bearing upon the development of creative thinking skills. Simonton (1989), in reviewing research on the developmental antecedents of creativity, noted that individuals who become eminent scientists are frequently the first born (Simonton, 1987; Roe, 1952a); suffer the loss of one parent by age 10 (Simonton, 1987; Roe, 1952a); and grow up in an environment with an abundance of intellectually enthralling materials, resulting in the acquisition, at an early age, of numerous stimulating hobbies (Simonton, 1987). Some of these characteristics are evident in the backgrounds of some of the eminent human action researchers included in this book.

Career experiences in other fields that are apparently unrelated, at a superficial level at least, to human action often significantly influence the subsequent career development of our eminent human action researchers. The early training of Kelso as a mathematics teacher, for example, may well have set in place the prerequisite analytical skills, if not the mode of thinking, that are reflected in his current theoretical contributions on the dynamics of motor learning and control. Similarly, Henry attributes his early personal experience as a Morse code operator as a contributing factor to his development of the memory drum theory (see Henry, 1981, and chapter 2 this volume). The analogies he used in the memory drum theory also reflect both a detailed personal knowledge of the operational mechanics of early computer hardware and the emerging technology of the era (cf. Gordon, 1989).

It appears that once a research interest is put in place, early success in getting research published serves as an important reinforcer. A number of expert human action researchers (e.g., Kelso, chapter 3, and Whiting, chapter 5) report that seeing their own work in print for the first time was an important stimulus for further research activity, an initially successful research experience having something of a self-perpetuating effect on continued research involvement.

What Types of Experimentation Do Expert Researchers Perform?

Chapter 1 emphasized that although the traditional model of the scientific method casts formal theory as an important precursor to experimentation, not all experimentation is in fact driven by theory. Rather, much experimentation proceeds in a bottom-up manner, with theory emerging from collected data rather than the reverse. As an additional alternative both theory and data may arise as secondary consequences, in some experimentation, of the desire to empirically test new methods and techniques. The autobiographical chapters reiterate the strong presence, even among expert researchers, of experimentation driven by data and by method, in addition to that driven by strong a priori theory.

Theory-Driven, Data-Driven, or Method-Driven Research? The type of experimentation favored by expert human action researchers is quite diverse, varying substantially among the small collection of expert researchers we have assembled for this book. Examples of research styles dominated by theory testing are provided by Kelso in motor learning and control and Roberts in sport psychology, although Kelso makes it clear in his chapter that in the early stages of his current research program (on the dynamics of human action), the theory being tested (especially with respect to the notion of nonlinear dissipative systems) was only very vaguely defined. The majority of our eminent human action researchers embark, at some time or another, on theory-driven research, but this is often equaled or surpassed in frequency by experimentation in which the original problem is only loosely defined and theory arises after rather than before data is collected. The autobiographies of Henry, Singer, and Carron, for example, reflect a strong mixture of top-down and data-driven experimentation. The abundance of data-driven research in the career of Henry is of particular interest given his principal recognition within the motor learning and control field as a theorist.

In the main, the theories tested by our eminent human action researchers have their origins in mainstream psychology (e.g., Singer's testing of early educational psychology theories in movement situations, Thomas's examination of neo-Piagetian theory, Roberts's examination of the McClelland-Atkinson and attributional theories of achievement motivation, and Rushall's testing of Skinnerian operant conditioning in sport settings), although Kelso is unique in taking his major theoretical premises from modern physics.* Key theoretical issues have been largely imported to the human action field from activities in other cognate disciplines rather than generated from original thinking within the field itself, giving rise to a dominance of "recipient paradigms," to use Wilberg's (1972) term. This is a pattern of development not unique to human action research, but one that dominates the genesis of new theory in virtually all branches of science. (This concept and its implications for expert experimentation will be considered in greater detail in the second section of this chapter.) The motor development field, in developing as something of a poor cousin to motor learning and control, has inherited many of the theories of the motor learning and control field. Sugden's testing of Fitts's (1954) law with subjects of different chronological age is a typical example of motor development's reliance on theory developments in the allied learning and control field.

The work of a number of eminent human action researchers (particularly Whiting and Keogh, and to a lesser extent Rarick and Sugden) is characterized primarily (and intentionally) by bottom-up (data-driven) experimentation strategies, the strategy that Whiting has described as "giving nature a prod and seeing how she reacted." Such research is frequently motivated by the need to solve practical problems or by the simple absence of sufficient basic factual information about the area of interest to support the postulation of any informed theory. Motor development provides many examples of the latter motive for data-driven research, and it is not surprising, given this outlook, to note a transition from data-driven to more theory-driven research, paralleling the career development of some of our expert motor development researchers, particularly Rarick and Thomas. For instance Thomas, in his chapter, notes that although he typically puts each study within some type of theoretical framework, the theory is often not what prompts the work in the first place.

The autobiographical account by Jerry Thomas (chapter 9) provides the only explicit example of method-driven research available from our sample of human action researchers, his dabbling with the technique of meta-analysis exemplifying the presence of a technique in search of a research program. It is clear from the Thomas example that, even with method as the initiating force, successful and important experimentation

---

*Kelso and other dynamic systems theorists (e.g., Turvey, Kugler, and Newell) seek increased explanatory power by appealing to theories from a more fundamental science (viz., physics), whereas the traditional approach within motor control has been to attempt to improve modeling by adding increased complexity and sophistication to favored views from cognitive psychology.

can be generated that may ultimately lead to theory and knowledge advancement in the field. In support of the notions introduced in chapter 1 (and summarized in Figure 1.1), it is apparent that experimentation is not a rigidly set sequence of procedures but rather a cycle of states that can be initiated from a number of different points. Although the progress of a field is inevitably linked to the development of good theory (i.e., theory that is capable of both succinctly summarizing the existing facts of the field and accurately predicting new events and directions), such a development may be achieved through forms of experimentation that are not explicitly theory driven. Because of this, successful experimenters display a diversity of approaches to experimentation. Expert researchers in the human action field, at least, are not characterized by their adoption of one common type of approach to experimentation, suggesting that theory-driven and data-driven research, in particular, should not be regarded as competing but rather as complementary modes of experimentation (Stelmach, 1987).

Level(s) of Analysis.   Just as expert experimenters in motor learning and control, motor development, and sport psychology do not select the same type of experimentation, they do not adopt a common level of analysis within their research work. Some expert experimenters rely on coarse-grained self-report measures (e.g., Roberts and Carron), some on behavioral/observational measures of movement (e.g., Keogh, Henry, and Sugden), and some on more detailed, fine-grained kinematic and kinetic analyses of movement process, as well as outcome variables (e.g., Kelso and Whiting). Level of analysis is constrained somewhat by technological development, and technological advances in biomechanics in particular have undoubtedly helped fuel the recent trend in motor learning and control and motor development toward more complex, fine-grained analyses that use kinematics to supplement traditional behavioral measures of movement outcome. This transition in level of analysis is evident in the work of Kelso and Whiting in motor learning and control, and of Thomas in motor development, and it is a necessary step to advance empirical tests of some of the emergent dynamic theories of motor learning and control. Similarly, although our expert sport and exercise psychology researchers use mainly self-report (Carron, Nideffer, and Roberts) and behavioral (Rushall) measures, there is also an increased use of fine-grained levels of analysis in this area. The electrophysiological work of Dan Landers and his colleagues (e.g., Hatfield, Landers, & Ray, 1987; Landers, Boutcher, & Wang, 1986b; Salazar, Landers, Petruzzello, Crews, & Kubitz, 1988) is a glowing example of the utilization of a micro rather than macro level of analysis in sport and exercise psychology and of a genuine attempt to use technological advances to overcome some of the inherent assumptions and limitations in the use of self-report and behavioral methodologies.

If expert experimenters share anything in common with respect to the level of analysis they select for their research work, it is their willingness to shift across levels of analysis in order to clarify and extend existing theoretical views. As Arbib (1972) noted with respect to the problem of understanding motor control,

> a scientist who works on any one level needs occasional forays both downward to find mechanisms for the functions studied, and upward to understand what role the studied function can play in the overall scheme of things. (p. 10)

The research work of motor developmentalist Lawrence Rarick (chapter 7) provides possibly the best example of a multilevel approach within our sample of experts; Rarick uses anthropometric and kinematic measures in conjunction with behavioral and self-report measures as a means of enhancing understanding of human growth and development. The value of multiple levels of analysis is that order and vital clues to important unitary control variables may be evident only at some levels of analysis and not at others. As a consequence, inclusion of measures sampling both macro and micro levels of human action is likely to be advantageous. As human movement studies develops as an area of study, and as collaborative work increases, the benefits of multiple levels of inquiry are likely to become more apparent and the use of such approaches is likely to become the norm.

Laboratory or Field Research?   As we noted in chapter 1, the researcher in selecting the appropriate setting in which to perform his or her experimentation is faced with a trade-off between the authenticity offered by the natural (field) setting and the direct control over variables of interest offered by the laboratory setting. Our expert human action researchers, typical of the broader population of movement scientists, have primarily opted for laboratory-based research in favor of field-based work, opting to sacrifice authenticity for added rigor and experimental control. Such research decisions are somewhat surprising, even paradoxical, given that the experimenters have expressed principal interests in understanding real-world phenomena and given that many of them were initially attracted to human action research through their own sporting, coaching, and teaching interests. The necessity for researchers in the human action field to be seen by their peers (particularly peers in experimental psychology) to be performing experimentation with the highest degree of rigor and control undoubtedly exerted a strong influence on the research setting decisions made by the researchers, particularly in the formative stages of their careers when the acceptability of their work to their peers was of paramount importance. Whiting and Rushall stand as exceptions; throughout their careers, these researchers have predominantly focused on experimentation upon (and observation of) natural skills performed in real-world settings. To some extent this field-based orientation has placed them outside the mainstream influences in their fields and forced them to struggle for acceptance of their work, particularly in the early stages of their careers. (Whiting's chapter reflects clearly upon this bias against field-based work, which dominated human action research, and experimental psychology in general, in the 1960s and 1970s.)

There are clear signs of a transition toward increased acceptance of, and indeed desire for, field-based research, and this transition is evident in the writings of a number of our expert experimenters (Kelso, Thomas, Carron, and Roberts). Such a transition has been fueled by a number of forces, including

- a general enlightenment in experimental psychology regarding the limitations of laboratory-based research (e.g., Gibbs, 1979; Neisser, 1976), recently reflected in the human action fields (e.g., Christina, 1987; Martens, 1979; Whiting, 1982);
- the emergence of theoretical views (especially those inspired by the ecological optics of J.J. Gibson [1979]) that highlight the necessity for ecological validity and the maintenance of perception and action in their normal, functional relationship; and
- technological advances that allow precise data collection to occur under noninvasive conditions.

Although a current focus upon experimentation in natural settings is obviously desirable in all branches of human action research in order to redress the historical imbalance toward laboratory-based research, the long-term progress of the motor learning and control, motor development, and sport and exercise psychology fields is likely dependent upon a balanced use of both laboratory-based and field-based experimentation (Christina, 1987). Testing key theories at a number of points throughout the laboratory-field continuum allows the experimenter to separate robust generic effects from situation-specific effects. Some of the autobiographies in this book reveal attempts to link field and laboratory research in a programmatic manner, and one might well expect increased diversity to characterize the research profiles of expert experimenters in the future. This linkage may occur in one of two possible ways. Keogh, for example, initially makes field-based observations and then uses them as a basis for later, more focused laboratory-based experimentation. In contrast, others (e.g., Thomas and Sugden), whose careers have been founded on laboratory-based research, are now headed clearly in the direction of testing the efficacy of existing theories under more natural field conditions.

Measurement and Data Analysis Preferences.   Like the choices of research design and style, which we examined earlier, the preference for particular data (and statistical) analytic methods turns out to be an individual one, not related in any direct way to experimenter expertise.

Although no single data analytic method either guarantees or precludes successful experimentation, it does appear that the more analytical methods a given experimenter is conversant and confident with, the better. As Platt (1964) suggested some years ago,

> Beware of the man of one method or one instrument, either experimental or theoretical. He tends to become method-oriented rather than problem-oriented; the method-oriented man is shackled. (p. 351)

Intense interest and specialization in measurement and data analytic methods often develop hand in glove with expertise in experimentation, often to the point where many eminent researchers become centrally interested in measurement issues per se, in some cases directing their focuses away from their original research interests. Ample examples of this are available from within the human action field, for example, Henry's preoccupation with error scores (Henry, 1959, 1974, 1975), Whiting's introduction to psychological research through hands-on experience with factor analysis, and Thomas's interest in meta-analysis (e.g., Thomas & French, 1985, 1986). It is interesting to note that this preoccupation with data analysis methods also occasionally extends to the development of specific instrumentation (Henry, Whiting, and Thomas all report on examples of this kind of activity as an essential part of the experimentation process for them) and to specific writings in the methods area (e.g., Thomas & Nelson, 1990). This general interest in measurement issues by some, but importantly not by all, of our expert researchers opposes the traditional view held by many experimentalists that statistical analysis is a means to an end rather than an end in itself. In some cases expert experimenters introduce new data analytic methods to their field (e.g., Rarick's introduction of multivariate methods to the motor development field), whereas in many other cases expert experimenters are happy to simply follow the traditional data analytic methods of the field.

Similarities Among Human Action Experimenters

Despite their superficial dissimilarity, those experimenters who have been successful in influencing the direction and orientation of their chosen research fields do share some common characteristics. We examine some of these in the next section.

Personality Characteristics of Successful Scientists

Detailed studies of successful researchers from other branches of science have revealed some common (and important) personality attributes (Simonton, 1988, 1989). Successful scientists, like other highly creative individuals, have cognitive styles that display extreme versatility and flexibility (White, 1931), wide categorization of disparate elements in grouping exercises (Cropley, 1967), and willingness to take intellectual risks (Cropley, 1967). The willingness to take risks appears to be particularly important; Stelmach (1987) noted that "scientists have an obligation to raise difficult questions, to take unpopular positions, and to accept intellectual risks if they are to create a significant body of research that opens new horizons for their contemporaries" (p. 24). Successful scientists have also been characterized by above-average intelligence (Cattell, 1963; Roe, 1952b), although, as Cox observed many years ago (Cox, 1926), exceptional intelligence does not guarantee success unless it is accompanied by high levels of achievement motivation and an extremely strong work ethic. Because immense productivity is a distinguishing attribute of scientific and other genius (Simonton, 1984), and because productivity is a positive function of the time allocated to scientific work* (Hargens, 1978; Simon, 1974), it is not surprising that productive and successful scientists are exceptionally hard working (McClelland, 1963) and persevering (Siegal & Zeigler, 1976, p. ix), displaying both "a driving absorption in their work" and a preference to work over virtually all other activities (Roe, 1952b, p. 25).

Although no direct evidence on personality characteristics, cognitive style, or intelligence was specifically collected from the sample of eminent human action researchers used in this book, ample evidence from the autobiographical reports indicates that our experts place similar importance upon hard work and perseverance as do successful experimenters in other branches of science. For example, Henry (chapter 2) in motor learning and control and Nideffer (chapter 11) in sport and exercise psychology both report that they were sufficiently motivated to overcome a number of barriers to their formal education and were so single-mindedly engrossed in their research that they worked happily without holidays or weekend breaks throughout the full duration of their PhD candidatures. Likewise, Kelso (chapter 3) alludes to the necessity for a "complete commitment" at various points in his career, and Singer (chapter 4), while describing the exhilaration of problem solving through science and his own addiction to experimentation, acknowledges the necessity to spend large amounts of time on the job in order to achieve success. Simonton (1989) argued that successful scientists display their unique combination of personality characteristics, cognitive styles, and work addictions because such characteristics facilitate the creativity needed in science to draw together apparently unrelated concepts and ideas to form new insights into old problems. Such a perspective on expertise is enlightening if expertise in experimentation is viewed in the context of introducing new ways of thinking into a given field.

---

*The reference to creative science as work seems appropriate given the extent of the work ethic evident in successful scientists (e.g., see Gruber, 1989; McClelland, 1961).

Expertise in Experimentation as the Ability to Introduce Paradigm Shifts

We noted in chapter 1, in discussing the history of science, that paradigm shifts (or what Kuhn, 1962, referred to as revolutionary science) are essential for the advancement of scientific fields. Publications that are labeled retrospectively as landmarks in the history of particular fields are those that substantially change the way of examining the major problems of the field (Diamond & Morton, 1978). It follows, therefore, that a key characteristic of the expert researcher is the ability to induce paradigm shifts (or cycles of revolutionary science) within a field of study. Expert researchers, we can argue, are such because they are capable of seeing and revealing new answers to old problems and they do so by introducing new paradigms of inquiry. The majority of researchers, in contrast to the experts, are primarily involved in experimentation more aligned with the causes of normal science and therefore rely upon the dominant paradigms established by the experts. It may well be, as Bernard (1927) remarked, that those "with a presentiment of new truths are rare in all sciences: most scientists develop and follow the ideas of a few others. Those who make discoveries are the promoters of new and fruitful ideas" (p. 13).

Within the human action research fields especially, and in science generally, changes in the dominant paradigm of a field of study (revolutionary science) are most often achieved through the adoption of paradigms and methods of study from other allied disciplines. Bartlett (1958) in his treatise on thinking noted the following:

> Over and over again the most outstanding scientific advances have been made when methods and instruments invented to deal with one set of problems have been taken over into areas with which they had little or nothing to do in their origin. (p. 161)

Likewise Koestler (1964), in discussing the genesis of scientific creativity, noted that "all decisive advances in the history of scientific thought can be described in terms of mental cross-fertilization between different disciplines" (p. 230).

Frequently, the importing of ideas from other fields of study is supplemented by the recognition of the significance of some older pieces of research that may have lay dormant for some time. The recent rediscovery and revitalization of the work of Bernstein in motor control (Bernstein, 1967; Whiting, 1984) is a good case in point.

There are numerous examples of researchers using paradigms from other fields to advance knowledge in the motor learning and control, motor development, and sport psychology fields. Particularly good examples of major paradigm changes introduced through adoption of the methods of other disciplines include the use of engineering and computer science methods in cognitive psychology and in turn in motor learning and control (via the information-processing model) and the recent adoptions of paradigms from theoretical physics in the understanding of motor control phenomena (e.g., Kelso & Scholtz, 1985; Kugler & Turvey, 1986; Schöner, Haken, & Kelso, 1986), as outlined in Kelso's chapter (chapter 3). (See Abernethy & Sparrow, 1992, for a review of these paradigm shifts in motor learning and control.)

Bartlett's (1958) observations on the use of ideas borrowed from other areas in inducing paradigm shifts have some important implications for how we should view the experimentation process and how we might expect young fields, like those involved in the understanding of human action, to develop. First, it is clear that *recipient* paradigms (i.e., paradigms borrowed from other fields), when used judiciously, are very important for knowledge advancement. It's also clear that views holding that paradigms developed within the field of study are more important than those developed in other disciplines (e.g., Wilberg, 1972) may be misleading. Clearly, however, the value of imported ideas and concepts needs to be closely evaluated on a situation-by-situation basis. As Bunge (1967) explained, exportable concepts (analogous to what we have termed recipient paradigms) to be fruitful "must cover at least the original concept and must suggest either fruitful new problems or must be assimilated by a scientific theory in the new field" (p. 109). Bunge warned that concepts from other fields "must not be used metaphorically or to give the appearance of a scientific approach or to cover conceptual indigence" (p. 109). An imported idea may actually retard conceptual development in an area if it "inhibits the search for new, emergent properties and laws rooted to those characterizing the lower levels but not identical with them" (Bunge, 1967, p. 111). Many (e.g., Carello et al., 1984; Kelso, 1986) argue, for example, that indiscriminate application of cybernetic concepts to motor control has restricted discovery of emergent properties of control inherent in the dynamics of muscle itself.

Second, it is clear that the process of science has an important social component to it, because contact with the research and writings of workers in other domains is an integral part of paradigm shifts and knowledge advance. (Carron also makes this point very clearly in chapter 10.) Bartlett (1958) suggested that "experimental thinking . . . is fundamentally cooperative, social, and cannot proceed far without the stimulus of outside contacts" (p. 123) and further that "perhaps all original ideas and developments come from contact of subject matter with different subject matter, of people with different people" (p. 147). Singer's contact with mainstream psychologists, the influence of the works of the physiologist Bernstein (1967) and the phenomenologist Ricoeur (1966) on Whiting, the impact of Skinner's (1938, 1950) works on Rushall, and Carron's indirect exposure to the work of Schutz (1966) on interpersonal compatibility are all examples of the kind of pervasive cross-disciplinary links that Bartlett regards as the basis of knowledge advancement. So important is social contact to knowledge advance that many modern students of scientific creativity (e.g., Gruber, 1989) view scientific work in the context of "networks of enterprise" that are of broad scope and that embrace many fields, such that progress in one field is a natural precursor to insight in another. The cross-fertilization of ideas that occurs in such networks is at the very heart of scientific revolution.

Third, given the importance of recipient paradigms for knowledge advance, it becomes inevitable that the genuine knowledge advance in a subject area through the cross-fertilization of ideas is accompanied by a concomitant breakdown of traditionally defined boundaries for given fields of study, the establishment of smaller specialized knowledge areas and units, and the establishment of more cross-disciplinary research problems and paradigms. Notable examples of such effects in the cognate areas include the establishment of psychophysiology from the union of psychology and physiology and the development of biochemistry as a hybrid of biology and chemistry. Similar evaporation of the traditional subdisciplinary boundaries has characterized the recent history and current research directions of the movement sciences (e.g., Brooks, 1981; Stelmach, 1987), although genuine interdisciplinary approaches to movement questions still remain uncommon. The importance of the relationship between the movement sciences and its allied disciplines has not escaped the attention of a number of our eminent human action researchers; Henry (1964, 1978), Rarick (1967), and Whiting (Brooke & Whiting, 1973) all have written at length about the disciplinary basis and status of the broader field of physical education and human movement studies.

Essential Characteristics of Experimenters Who Induce Paradigm Shifts

Some important observations on the characteristics of expert experimentation can also be gleaned from recognition of the roles that imported (recipient) knowledge and concepts play in inducing the paradigm shifts and revolutionary science that are essential for the advance of the field. Clearly, the successful experimenter must be able to recognize and draw generalities across diverse fields of study. To quote again from Bartlett (1958),

> The most important of all conditions of originality in experimental thinking is a capacity to detect overlap and agreement between groups of facts and fields of study which have not before been effectively combined and to bring these groups into experimental contact. (p. 162)

and

The most important feature of original experimental thinking is the discovery of overlap and agreement where formerly only isolation and difference were recognized. (p. 136)

Frequently, commonalities across fields are apparent to no one initially but can be easily described and understood once the relationship is demonstrated (see also Kelso, chapter 3 this volume).

The Importance of Knowledge and Experience in Other Fields. An experimenter's ability to recognize generalities across disparate bodies of knowledge and to import outside ideas into new problem areas is a function both of the breadth and depth of the experimenter's formal educational training and of his or her skills development and experience in other apparently unrelated spheres and trades. Eclecticism of knowledge and experience is clearly important, often to the point where innovative scientists frequently bridge two or more fields without really belonging to any of them. For this reason, professional and sociocultural marginality is frequently an important predictor of creativity in a number of scientific fields (Campbell, 1960; Simonton, 1989). (Gleick's 1987 chronicle of the development of modern chaos theory, for example, refers to many such scientists, seen by both the disciplines of mathematics and physics as outsiders.)

One can easily postulate from the information available on the backgrounds of some of our eminent human action researchers how their formative experiences in other fields may have helped create the mental sets upon which their later theoretical contributions to human action research were based. As noted earlier in this chapter, Henry's early experience as a Morse code operator and Kelso's background as a mathematics teacher may well have provided important knowledge about the theory and practice of other areas of science and technology that these researchers could then apply to the understanding of motor control phenomena. The adoption of paradigms from other fields of study is not simply a passive process but one that requires expert experimenters to use their unique knowledge of their own subject matter to make appropriate situation-specific modifications and to perform tests of recipient paradigms' applicability in their adopted settings.

The Essential Knowledge Bases for Expertise. Being able to make the link between an existing problem and the methods and paradigms of other disciplines requires not only an intimate knowledge of the specific content of the area under examination but also an understanding of the deeper structure of the subject matter in a number of areas. This attunement to "deep" structure (underlying laws, principles, and theoretical commonalities) is a characteristic of expert problem solving that is common to a number of cognitive activities (e.g., Chiesi, Spilich, & Voss, 1979; Elstein, Shulman, & Sprafka, 1978; Hunter, 1968; Larkin, McDermott,

Simon, & Simon, 1980; McKeithen, Reitman, Rueter, & Hirtle, 1981; Schoenfeld & Herrmann, 1982). In other fields, this transition from reliance on the superficial (surface) characteristics of the data available to reliance on deeper characteristics of the problem itself appears to occur as a consequence of extensive task-specific practice and experience (e.g., J.R. Thomas, French, Thomas, & Gallagher, 1988). Not surprisingly, commonality exists between the kind of thinking demanded of expert scholars (in searching for the deeper structure of knowledge) and the kind of knowledge progression (from facts to laws) demanded by science.

It is useful for comparative purposes, therefore, to consider successful experimentation as another example of skilled problem-solving activity, and a useful schema for considering problem-solving activity is through the various forms of knowledge development and representation variously described by J.R. Anderson (1976, 1982), Brown (1975; Brown & DeLoache, 1978), Chi (1978, 1981; Chi & Glaser, 1980; Chi, Glaser, & Farr, 1988), and Norman and Shallice (1985).* Although consideration of these various knowledge forms introduces yet another ontology for cognitive psychology, it is nevertheless a very enlightening perspective from which to examine the nature of expertise.

Experts in a range of cognitive tasks have been shown to possess greater declarative, procedural, strategic, and metacognitive skills than appropriately matched novices. Declarative knowledge refers to knowledge about factual information (e.g., specifics about key papers or findings in a researcher's specialized field of study). Procedural knowledge involves knowing how to solve problems within one's specific field of study. Both declarative knowledge and procedural knowledge are considered to be domain specific, pertaining to facts, rules, or principles that are relatively "local" in nature. Strategic knowledge refers to knowledge of more global, general rules and principles applicable across a range of different domains (e.g., knowledge of the applicability of general notions and issues, such as the nature-nurture issue or the authenticity-control trade-off in experimentation, that hold across different specific bodies of knowledge and fields of study).

A wide range of evidence drawn from examination of knowledge related to topics such as chess (Chase & Simon, 1973; Chi, 1978), bridge (Engle & Bukstel, 1978), and baseball (Chiesi et al., 1979; Spilich, Vesonder, Chiesi, & Voss, 1979) indicates that the development of great amounts of declarative knowledge is an essential characteristic of cognitive expertise. This growth in declarative knowledge that accompanies growing expertise is usually viewed in terms of an expanding propositional network (J.R.

---

*I am indebted to Ted Wall and Jerry Thomas for initially drawing my attention to this body of literature. Not surprisingly the viewpoint presented here is influenced strongly by their work (e.g., J.R. Thomas et al., 1986; J.R. Thomas, French, Thomas, & Gallagher, 1988; Wall, 1986; Wall, McClements, Bouffard, Findlay, & Taylor, 1985).

Thomas, French, Thomas, & Gallagher, 1988). Knowing more factual information implies the acquisition of more concepts (or nodes or chunks; Norman & Shallice, 1985), the acquisition of a greater number of features used to unambiguously specify and define each feature, and the development of a greater network of interconcept links (Chi & Glaser, 1980; Murphy & Wright, 1984).

The development of expertise in cognitive tasks is also related to the development of greater procedural knowledge, experts having greater knowledge than novices on how to go about solving domain-specific problems (e.g., Adelson, 1984; Chi, Feltovich, & Glaser, 1981). The importance of procedural knowledge development may well surpass that of factual knowledge development for the cognitive activities that are required of scientists. Procedural knowledge development is characterized by the production of a large range of generalized conditional statements that specify the relationship between important domain features. In many cases, this procedural knowledge development appears to occur somewhat spontaneously and subconsciously and, therefore, often cannot be reported by the expert. This subconscious development of links between existing knowledge is typical of the "aha" phenomenon frequently reported by scientists in arriving at new hypotheses or solving old problems. As J.R. Thomas et al. (1986) reported,

> experts possess a rich semantic network of declarative knowledge and a system of procedural knowledge that allows them to form an abstract plan for solving problems with greater ease than novices, even though the experts may be unaware of the detailed processes by which the procedural knowledge was used in the solution process. (p. 265)

These declarative and procedural knowledge characteristics of cognitive expertise are clearly congruent with some of the demands of the experimentation process as identified in chapter 1. However, these forms of knowledge alone, although they seem necessary for successful experimentation, are insufficient to support experimentation of the type needed to move beyond normal science and induce paradigm shifts within a field of study. Such expert experimentation seems to demand, in addition,

- a richly developed strategic knowledge base (as an essential requirement for introducing theories, methods, and paradigms of research from other fields to the immediate problems posed within the researcher's specialist field); and
- well-advanced metacognitive skills (to support experimenters in their performances of the mental experiments necessary for the assessment and design of potentially innovative paradigms and to help experimenters monitor and evaluate whether their ongoing work is progressive or recessive).

The importance of a well-developed knowledge base is implicit in the following statement of the goals of science by Kroll (1971).

> Although a science is concerned with the production and accumulation of knowledge, it is more concerned with discovering relationships among such data and with developing an understanding of broader and broader systems. Accumulation of a thousand new facts is good, but formulation of a general principle that can explain all the facts present and the thousands of new facts likely to come from the content domain is even better. (p. 206)

The development of effective strategic knowledge depends on the existence of a strong procedural knowledge base, which, in turn, is formed from the foundation of a strong body of declarative knowledge (J.R. Anderson, 1982; Chi, 1981). Gains in the global strategic knowledge are, therefore, contingent upon the pyramidal type development of both the domain-specific procedural and the declarative knowledge forms (Figure 14.1). Viewed in this way, with strategic knowledge development seen as an essential condition for expertise in experimentation, the knowledge-based approach is very useful in explaining two key observations about the progress of knowledge in specific fields, such as that concerned with the understanding of human action. First, the pyramidal nature of knowledge development means that by definition fewer experimenters reach the stage of operating on the basis of strategic knowledge rather than procedural and in turn declarative knowledge. This leaves the great majority of researchers to practice normal science rather than revolutionary science and leaves only a relative minority of the total pool of experimenters capable of inducing paradigm shifts. Second, this concept can also explain why many of those experimenters who have played a part in inducing paradigm shifts within a field have spent considerable time in the early part of their research careers pursuing normal science

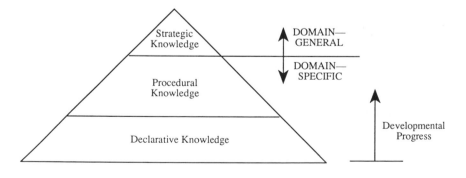

Figure 14.1   A heuristic for the consideration of knowledge development by the expert researcher.

and following traditional lines of research (Kelso is a good example within the human action field). The early pursuit of traditional research topics is encouraged by procedural knowledge competence, and it is only with the acquisition and maturation of more global, non-domain-specific, strategic knowledge that experimenters are able to introduce the recipient paradigms from other fields necessary to induce paradigm shifts within their own specialist fields.

Implications for Postgraduate Training. The academic preparation the researcher receives, as both an undergraduate and graduate, has a strong influence on the researcher's potential to make a substantial impact on the field. Given what we have just discussed about the knowledge base of expert experimenters, it is clear that academic preparation of the researcher in the field of human action should ideally include a strong declarative knowledge base, as the foundation for the development of strong higher order knowledge in both domain-specific and general areas. This should include not only some detailed exposure to the content and methods of relevant mainstream disciplines (especially psychology and physiology) but also, arguably, some movement-skill-specific knowledge (after J.R. Thomas et al., 1986). The preparation of expert experimenters needs to include not only exposure to detailed domain-specific information but also broad exposure to other potentially overlapping fields of scientific endeavor. This exposure to the methods, theories, and paradigms of other areas allows expert researchers both to cross the boundaries created by different levels of analysis of the same problem and to import recipient paradigms from other fields that allow old problems to be viewed from new (and we hope more enlightening) perspectives (see also Canic, 1988).

Stelmach and Diggles (1982), in discussing conceptual development in the motor control field, indicate that a broad educational background is necessary to develop the skills needed to cross different levels of analysis.

> To successfully accomplish the interaction between levels of inquiry and disciplines, individuals will require a broader background in a number of areas. A functional understanding of key concepts from a number of disciplines studying the biological and behavioral determinants of movement is necessary . . . behavioral models have changed in accordance with discoveries in supporting disciplines, and the motor control area will take advantage of progress in related disciplines. (p. 100)

Glassford (1987) makes a similar point in concluding his critique of the specialization-fragmentation debate in graduate education for the movement sciences (Harris & Park, 1987). Glassford suggests that

> It is not a blind allegiance to one specific world view and its concomitant methodologies that is important but an ability to think creatively

and to have a sound conceptual base on which to build a world view.
(p. 295)

Exposure to a broad range of disciplines is an important starting point
for the development of the eclecticism needed by the expert researcher
(Dunnett, 1966). Acquiring a broad knowledge of the methods and perspectives of different fields may be one of the best ways for a researcher
to avoid becoming shackled to single perspectives and unitary paradigms
(Landers, 1983).

Strategies Expert Experimenters Use to Enhance
Their Abilities to Make Important Findings
and Induce Paradigm Shifts

Constant Exposure to New Ideas.   As we have seen, key advances in
specific fields of knowledge often arise when expert experimenters adopt
and adapt the methods and paradigms of other areas to solve specific
problems within their own research fields. To make the links needed for
such paradigmatic transfer, the expert experimenter must have not only
broad initial training and interests and higher order development of
strategic knowledge skills but also constant exposure to new ideas. This
constant refreshment of the knowledge pool seems to be essential to the
advancement of knowledge in any field of study, and it implicates
heavily the necessity for knowledge exchange through such avenues as
conferences, study leaves, interdisciplinary workshops, and especially
exposure to new colleagues and postgraduate students. A number of the
eminent researchers assembled in this book (e.g., Kelso, Keogh, and
Whiting) explicitly acknowledge the role that colleagues from outside
their immediate discipline areas play in influencing their thinking and
their approaches to problems in the human action field. Many of our
expert experimenters (e.g., Carron, Singer, and Thomas) also accredit
substantial portions of their success to having access to a constant pool
of talented graduate students who provide new ideas and perspectives.
This is a situation that some eminent researchers in mainstream psychology (e.g., Cattell, 1984) also acknowledge as an integral part of their
achievements in science.

Predicting Fruitful Lines of Inquiry.   Once an experimenter becomes
established in a research position, a key prerequisite for ongoing success
appears to be the ability to predict fruitful lines of change (i.e., new
research directions), so as to maintain an active, progressive program of
research over an extended period of time.* As Bartlett (1958) noted in his
classical treatise of the essential characteristics of experimental thinking,

---

*It is worth noting, as a general rule, that eminent experimenters are typically characterized
more by research programs than by the single outstanding acts of experimentation.

an experimenter must "know" what dimensions of change it is likely to be worth his while to select for experimental control. This seems to demand some "superior sensitivity" to "dead ends"—if the experiments get more or less near them—and to the proximity of openings so many, so varied, and so general that if he proceeds he is likely to wander aimlessly. (p. 162)

Judging whether a particular research paradigm is progressive or degenerative (Lakatos, 1970a, 1970b; Lakatos & Zahar, 1975; Zahar, 1973) requires, among other things, the following:

- Awareness of the history of the field as a means of predicting future directions
- Finely attuned sensitivity to dead ends (i.e., nonproductive research directions)
- Willingness to change and/or abandon a line of work or a paradigm in which a substantial amount of time, energy, resources, and emotion has been invested (e.g., see Martens, 1987)
- Willingness to pursue innovative (risky) lines of inquiry that differ from the tried and proven approaches to the subject matter
- Willingness to learn new approaches and new bodies of literature even when these were either nonexistent or apparently unimportant at the time of the experimenter's education (e.g., see Whiting, chapter 5, this volume)

How then might expert experimenters go about distinguishing between progressive and degenerative research programs? According to Lakatos (1970a, 1970b) a progressive program of experimentation is one that involves historical change that not only allows anomalous results to be adequately accommodated but also successfully predicts the occurrence of novel events. A degenerative program of experimentation occurs when modifications to theory and paradigm are made specifically to accommodate troublesome data within the existing dominant paradigm and provide no additional predictive value. Lakatos (1970a, 1970b) suggested a particular theory and paradigm should be abandoned when additional ad hoc modifications are unlikely to allow degenerative programs of research to become more progressive, whereas others (e.g., Kendler, 1981, pp. 147-148) have argued that the criterion for abandonment needs to be more complex than simply the extension of predictability.

In practice the decision to abandon a given theory or line of research is often made on grounds other than logic. The personality of and time invested by the researcher in pursuing a particular theoretical perspective seem to be particularly important—the more stubborn the researcher or the more time he or she has spent examining a given theory, the lower the probability of a rapid abandonment (Kuhn, 1962). Kendler (1981) noted, however, that neither choice (persistence or abandonment) creates any long-term obstacles to the progress of knowledge. Persistence may provide information about the value of new revisions to old theories, whereas abandonment serves as a general notice of the unsatisfactory nature of the old theoretical position. As Kendler (1981) observed, "the choice to abandon indicates that a former adherent has reached the considered judgment that his research program is hopelessly degenerated, and therefore the scientific community is advised to expend no further effort to salvage it" (p. 149).

One way that expert experimenters avoid the disappointment associated with the pursuit of degenerative lines of research and the disappointment of abandonment is to pursue many clues and lines of inquiry simultaneously. Expert experimenters improve their chances of making meaningful progress by having multiple research tacks that run in parallel, even though many of these lines may ultimately prove fruitless and must be discarded. An experimenter can make progress along some lines of inquiry when other lines reach an impasse and become dormant (cf. Gruber, 1989). This research strategy usually requires the experimenter to be in a well-established research position and to utilize secondhand data collection via postgraduate students or paid research assistants—a strategy that paradoxically places the researcher further and further from the original subjects and data as he or she becomes more successful (Cohen, 1977, p. 334).

A number of examples of multiple research interests are apparent among the autobiographies provided by the expert human action researchers in this book (e.g., Singer, chapter 4, provides a good example), and the use of multiple research programs is advocated as a discovery strategy by a number of human action researchers, particularly in the sport and exercise psychology field (e.g., Feltz, 1987; Landers, 1983). The design and administration of multiple research programs can only be effective, however, if the researcher is highly motivated and prepared to accept the elevated work load associated with such an undertaking—characteristics we have already seen as common among successful scientists and successful experimenters in the human action field.

Another strategy used by expert experimenters to improve their chances of research success is to perform "mind experiments." Many expert experimenters are able to think through potential experiments from the design stage through to data collection, analysis, and interpretation of possible results; this is a means of determining if a particular line of research is viable without actually physically undertaking the experiment (Bartlett, 1958). Siegal and Zeigler (1976), commenting on the autobiographical accounts of research by experts in psychology contained within their edited book, noted that although

the popular notion of just how science is done may be far more elegant . . . almost all of the contributors to this book have commented that they first performed little "thought experiments," tried out an idea on their children or spouses, or ran simple, informal tests. (p. x)

Such mental experimentation relies on the expert experimenter's knowledge and awareness of his or her own style of thinking and level of knowing—what is frequently referred to as metacognitive knowledge (Brown & DeLoache, 1978).

The net effect of running parallel lines of experimentation, including mind experiments, is that the expert experimenter increases the total number of experiments conducted in a given unit of time. This may well be important not only in terms of sheer productivity but also because the more experiments that are conducted and options that are examined, the greater is the probability that the experimenter will make an important discovery. Simonton (1989), drawing heavily on the work of Campbell (1960), argued that creativity comes largely from random processes, and as a consequence the expert experimenter, by employing strategies that increase the number of experiments that are conducted, also improves his or her chance of discovering something of importance.

The Role of Serendipity.   The preceding discussion suggests that serendipity may play a major role in discovery in science, and indeed the metascience literature abounds with anecdotes concerning the role of chance in pivotal scientific discoveries (e.g., Cannon, 1940; Koestler, 1964; Mach, 1896). Fortune undoubtedly plays a key role in the success of a number of experiments and programs of research (see Kelso, Thomas, and Roberts in chapters 3, 9, and 12 of this volume for examples of serendipitous findings or events in their careers that have led to fruitful research paradigms in the human action field), although perhaps it should be more appropriately regarded as opportunism (Bartlett, 1958, p. 131). As Siegal and Zeigler (1976) observed from their sample of eminent psychologists, "What is required, evidently, is not only luck, but an awareness that something significant has been found and a willingness to wonder about it" (p. x).

Of course, nothing is ever entirely new in the field of science, and history frequently reveals that many pivotal findings that change the direction of research in a particular field have been made earlier but their significance was not appreciated at the time. Kelso (chapter 3) recounts one such occurrence in the human action field, and the recent emergence of chaos theory (chronicled in Gleick's 1987 text) provides many such examples of this phenomenon. Louis Pasteur undoubtedly struck at the heart of the problem of expertise, education, and scientific progress, in general, when he noted many years ago that "chance only favors the mind which is prepared" (Vallery-Radot, 1911, p. 76). It is our hope that the collective contents of this book may, in some small way, aid in preparing the minds of the forthcoming generation of human action researchers, so that our knowledge of human action may be meaningfully advanced through experimentation.

References

Abernethy, B., & Sparrow, W.A. (1992). The rise and fall of dominant paradigms in motor behaviour research. In J.J. Summers (Ed.), *Approaches to the study of motor control and learning* (pp. 3-45). Amsterdam: North-Holland.

Adams, J.A. (1971). A closed-loop theory of motor learning. *Journal of Motor Behavior,* **3,** 111-150.

Adams, J.A. (1987). Historical review and appraisal of research on the learning, retention, and transfer of human motor skills. *Psychological Bulletin,* **101,** 41-74.

Adelson, B. (1984). When novices surpass experts: The difficulty of a task may increase with expertise. *Journal of Experimental Psychology: Learning, Memory and Cognition,* **10,** 483-495.

Agnew, N.M., & Pyke, S.W. (1969). *The science game.* Englewood Cliffs, NJ: Prentice Hall.

Alderson, G.J.K., & Whiting, H.T.A. (1974). Prediction of linear motion. *Human Factors,* **16,** 495-502.

Ames, C. (1984). Competitive, cooperative, and individualistic goal structure: A cognitive-motivational analysis. In R. Ames & C. Ames (Eds.), *Research on motivation in education. Vol. 1: Student motivation* (pp. 177-208). New York: Academic Press.

Ames, C. (1992). Achievement goals, motivational climate, and motivational processes. In G.C. Roberts (Ed.), *Motivation in sport and exercise* (pp. 161-176). Champaign, IL: Human Kinetics.

Ames, L.B. (1937). The sequential patterning of prone progression in the human infant. *Genetic Psychology Monographs,* **19,** 409-460.

Anderson, J.R. (1976). *Language, memory, and thought.* Hillsdale, NJ: Erlbaum.

Anderson, J.R. (1982). Acquisition of cognitive skill. *Psychological Review,* **89,** 369-406.

Anderson, W.G. (1899). Studies in the effects of physical training. *American Physical Education Review,* **4,** 265-278.

Arbib, M. (1972). *The metaphorical brain*. New York: Wiley-Interscience.

Argyris, C. (1975). Dangers in applying results from experimental social psychology. *American Psychologist, 30*, 469-485.

Atkinson, J.W. (1957). Motivational determinants of risk-taking behaviors. *Psychological Review, 64*, 359-372.

Atkinson, J.W. (1964). *An introduction to motivation*. Princeton, NJ: Van Nostrand.

Bachrach, A.J. (1965). *Psychological research* (2nd ed.). New York: Random House.

Ball, J.R., & Carron, A.V. (1976). The influence of team cohesion and participation motivation upon performance success in intercollegiate ice hockey. *Canadian Journal of Applied Sport Sciences, 1*, 271-275.

Bandura, A. (1977). Self-efficacy: Toward a unifying theory of personality change. *Psychological Review, 84*, 191-215.

Bartlett, F.C. (1958). *Thinking: An experimental and social study*. London: Unwin University Books.

Bayley, N. (1935). Development of motor abilities during the first three years. *Monographs of the Society for Research in Child Development, 1*, 1-26.

Beek, P.J., & Meijer, O.G. (1988). On the nature of 'the' motor-action controversy. In O.G. Meijer & K. Roth (Eds.), *Complex movement behaviour: 'The' motor-action controversy* (pp. 157-185). Amsterdam: North-Holland.

Belmont, J.M., & Butterfield, E.C. (1969). The relation of short-term memory to development and intelligence. In L. Lipsitt & H.W. Reese (Eds.), *Advances in child development and behavior* (Vol. 4). New York: Academic Press.

Bender, P.R. (1976). *A developmental explanation of motor behavior: A neo-Piagetian interpretation*. Unpublished doctoral dissertation, Florida State University, Tallahassee.

Berliner, D.C. (1986). In pursuit of the expert pedagogue. *Educational Researcher, 15*(7), 5-13.

Bernard, C. (1927). *An introduction to the study of experimental medicine* (H.E. Greene, Trans.). New York: Macmillan.

Bernstein, N. (1967). *The coordination and regulation of movements*. Oxford, UK: Pergamon Press.

Bizzi, E., Polit, A., & Morasso, P. (1976). Mechanisms underlying achievement of final head position. *Journal of Neurophysiology, 39*, 435-444.

Bloor, D. (1971). Two paradigms of scientific knowledge? *Science Studies, 1*, 101-115.

Boring, E.G. (1954). The nature and history of experimental control. *The American Journal of Psychology, 67*, 573-589.

Brawley, L.R., Carron, A.V., & Widmeyer, W.N. (1987). Assessing the cohesion of sport teams: Validity of the Group Environment Questionnaire. *Journal of Sport Psychology, 9*, 275-294.

Brawley, L.R., & Roberts, G.C. (1984). Attribution in sport: Research founda-tions, characteristics, and limitations. In J.M. Silva & R.S. Weinberg (Eds.), *Psychological foundations of sport* (pp. 197-213). Champaign, IL: Human Kinetics.

Broadbent, D.E. (1971). *Relation between theory and application in psychology.* (Tech. Rep. No. 879/71). Cambridge, UK: Medical Research Council, Applied Psychology Unit.

Bronfenbrenner, U. (1977). Toward an experimental ecology of human development. *American Psychologist, 32,* 513-531.

Brooke, J.D., & Whiting, H.T.A. (Eds.) (1973). *Human movement—a field of study.* London: Henry Kimpton.

Brooks, G.A. (Ed.) (1981). *Perspectives on the academic discipline of physical education.* Champaign, IL: Human Kinetics.

Brown, A.L. (1975). The development of memory: Knowing, knowing how to know and knowing about knowing. In H.W. Reese (Ed.), *Advances in child development and behavior* (Vol. 10). New York: Academic Press.

Brown, A.L., & DeLoache, J.S. (1978). Skills, plans, and self-regulation. In R.S. Siegler (Ed.), *Children's thinking: What develops?* (pp. 3-35). Hills-dale, NJ: Erlbaum.

Brunswick, E. (1952). The conceptual framework of psychology. *International Encyclopedia of Unified Sciences, 6,* 659-751.

Bryan, W.L., & Harter, N. (1897). Studies in the physiology and psychology of telegraphic language. *Psychological Review, 4,* 27-53.

Bryan, W.L., & Harter, N. (1899). Studies on the telegraphic language: The acquisition of a hierarchy of habits. *Psychological Review, 6,* 345-375.

Bunge, M. (1967). *Scientific research I: The search for system.* Berlin: Springer-Verlag.

Burnside, L.H. (1927). Coordination in the locomotion of infants. *Genetic Psychology Monographs, 2,* 279-372.

Burton, D. (1983). *Evaluation of goal setting training on selected cognitions and performance of collegiate swimmers.* Unpublished doctoral dissertation, University of Illinois, Urbana-Champaign.

Campbell, D.T. (1960). Blind variation and selective retention in creative thought as in other knowledge processes. *Psychological Review, 67,* 380-400.

Canic, M.J. (1988). The value of a multidisciplinary education for the student of physical performance. In F.A. Carre (Ed.), *Towards the 21st century* (pp. 275-278). Proceedings of the 30th ICHPER World Congress and the 34th CAHPER Conference. Vancouver, BC: School of Physical Education and Recreation, University of British Columbia.

Cannon, W.B. (1940). The role of chance in discovery. *Scientific Monthly, 50,* 204-209.

Carello, C., Turvey, M.T., Kugler, P.N., & Shaw, R.E. (1984). Inadequacies in the computer metaphor. In M. Gazzaniga (Ed.), *Handbook of cognitive neuroscience* (pp. 229-248). New York: Plenum Press.

Carr, D. (1981). Professionalisation in education and physical education: A reply to David Best. *British Journal of Educational Studies, 29*, 152-158.

Carron, A.V. (1968). Motor performance under stress. *Research Quarterly, 39*, 463-469.

Carron, A.V. (1969a). Discrete trial motor learning: Influence of practice on individual differences and intra-individual variability. *Perceptual and Motor Skills, 28*, 827-831.

Carron, A.V. (1969b). Performance and learning in a discrete motor task under massed versus distributed practice. *Research Quarterly, 40*, 481-489.

Carron, A.V. (1969c). Physical fatigue and motor learning. *Research Quarterly, 40*, 682-686.

Carron, A.V. (1971a). *Laboratory experiments in motor learning.* Englewood Cliffs, NJ: Prentice Hall.

Carron, A.V. (1971b). Motor performance and response consistency as a function of age. *Journal of Motor Behavior, 3*, 105-109.

Carron, A.V. (1980). *Social psychology of sport.* Ithaca, NY: Mouvement.

Carron, A.V. (1981). *An experiential approach to the social psychology of sport.* Ithaca, NY: Mouvement.

Carron, A.V. (1982). Cohesiveness in sport groups: Interpretations and considerations. *Journal of Sport Psychology, 4*, 123-138.

Carron, A.V. (1984). *Motivation: Implications for coaching and teaching.* London, ON: Spodym.

Carron, A.V. (1988). *Group dynamics in sport: Theoretical and practical issues.* London, ON: Spodym.

Carron, A.V., & Bailey, D.A. (1973). A longitudinal examination of speed of reaction and speed of movement in young boys 7 to 13 years. *Human Biology, 45*, 663-681.

Carron, A.V., & Bailey, D.A. (1974). Strength development in boys from 10 through 16 years. *Monograph for the Society for Research in Child Development,* November, Serial No. 157, No. 4.

Carron, A.V., & Bennett, B.B. (1977). Compatibility in the coach-athlete dyad. *Research Quarterly, 48*, 671-679.

Carron, A.V., & Chelladurai, P. (1981). Cohesion as a factor in sport performance. *International Review of Sport Sociology, 1*, 2-41.

Carron, A.V., & Leavitt, J.L. (1968a). The effects of practice on individual differences and intra-variability in a motor skill. *Research Quarterly, 39*, 470-474.

Carron, A.V., & Leavitt, J.L. (1968b). Individual differences in two motor learning tasks under massed practice. *Perceptual and Motor Skills, 27*, 499-504.

Carron, A.V., & Marteniuk, R.G. (1970). An examination of the selection of criterion scores for the study of motor learning and retention. *Journal of Motor Behavior, 2*, 239-244.

Carron, A.V., & Morford, R.W. (1968). Anxiety, stress, and motor learning. *Perceptual and Motor Skills, 27,* 507-511.

Carron, A.V., Widmeyer, W.N., & Brawley, L.R. (1985). The development of an instrument to assess cohesion in sport teams: The Group Environment Questionnaire. *Journal of Sport Psychology, 7,* 244-266.

Castine, S.C., & Roberts, G.C. (1974). Modeling in the socialization process of the black athlete. *International Review of Sociology, 9,* 59-73.

Cattell, R.B. (1963). The personality and motivation of the researcher from measurements of contemporaries and from biography. In C.W. Taylor & F. Barron (Eds.), *Scientific creativity* (pp. 119-131). New York: Wiley.

Cattell, R.B. (1984). The voyage of a laboratory, 1928-1984. *Multivariate Behavioral Research, 19,* 121-174.

Chalmers, A.F. (1982). *What is this thing called science?* (2nd ed.). Brisbane, Australia: University of Queensland Press.

Chase, W.G., & Simon, H.A. (1973). Perception in chess. *Cognitive Psychology, 4,* 55-81.

Chelladurai, P., & Carron, A.V. (1978). *Leadership* (CAHPER Sociology of Sport Monograph Series). Ottawa, ON: Canadian Association for Health, Physical Education and Recreation.

Chi, M.T.H. (1976). Short-term memory limitations in children: Capacity or processing deficits? *Memory and Cognition, 4,* 559-572.

Chi, M.T.H. (1978). Knowledge structures and memory development. In R.S. Siegler (Ed.), *Children's thinking: What develops?* (pp. 73-105). Hillsdale, NJ: Erlbaum.

Chi, M.T.H. (1981). Knowledge development and memory performance. In M.P. Friedman, J.P. Das, & N. O'Connor (Eds.), *Intelligence and learning* (pp. 221-229). New York: Plenum Press.

Chi, M.T.H., Feltovich, P.J., & Glaser, R. (1981). Categorization and representation of physics problems by experts and novices. *Cognitive Science, 5,* 121-152.

Chi, M.T.H., & Glaser, R. (1980). The measurement of expertise: Analysis of the development of knowledge and skill as a basis for assessing achievement. In E.L. Baker & E.S. Quellmely (Eds.), *Educational testing and evaluation* (pp. 37-47). Beverly Hills, CA: Sage.

Chi, M.T.H., Glaser, R., & Farr, M.J. (Eds.) (1988). *The nature of expertise.* Hillsdale, NJ: Erlbaum.

Chiesi, H.L., Spilich, G.J., & Voss, J.F. (1979). Acquisition of domain related information in relation to high and low domain knowledge. *Journal of Verbal Learning and Verbal Behavior, 18,* 257-273.

Chissom, B.S., Thomas, J.R., & Collins, D.G. (1974). Relationships among perceptual-motor measures and their correlations with academic readiness for preschoolers. *Perceptual and Motor Skills, 39,* 467-473.

Chorkawy, A.L. (1982). *The effects of cognitive strategies on the performance of female swimmers*. Unpublished master's thesis, Lakehead University, Thunder Bay, ON.

Christina, R.W. (1987). Motor learning: Future lines of research. In M.J. Safrit & H.M. Eckert (Eds.), *The cutting edge in physical education and exercise science research* (pp. 26-41). Champaign, IL: Human Kinetics.

Christina, R.W. (1989). Whatever happened to applied research in motor learning? In J.S. Skinner, C.B. Corbin, D.M. Landers, P.E. Martin, & C.L. Wells (Eds.), *Future directions in exercise and sport science research* (pp. 411-422). Champaign, IL: Human Kinetics.

Clark, C.E. (1966). *Random numbers in uniform and normal distributions*. San Francisco: Chandler.

Clarke, H.H. (1971). *Physical and motor tests in the Medford boys' growth study*. Englewood Cliffs, NJ: Prentice Hall.

Clogston, A.M. (1987). Applied research: Key to innovation. *Science, 235*, 12-13.

Cohen, D. (1977). *Psychologists on psychology*. London: Ark Paperbacks.

Cohen, L. (1971). Synchronous bimanual movements performed by homologous and non-homologous muscles. *Perceptual and Motor Skills, 32*, 639-644.

Connolly, K.J. (Ed.) (1970a). *Mechanisms of motor skill development*. London: Academic Press.

Connolly, K.J. (1970b). Response speed, temporal sequencing and information processing in children. In K.J. Connolly (Ed.), *Mechanisms of motor skill development* (pp. 161-188). New York: Academic Press.

Connolly, K.J. (1986). A perspective on motor development. In M.G. Wade & H.T.A. Whiting (Eds.), *Motor development in children: Aspects of coordination and control* (pp. 3-21). Dordrecht, Netherlands: Martinus Nijhoff.

Corder, W.O. (1966). Effects of physical education on the intellectual, physical and social development of educable mentally retarded boys. *Exceptional Children, 32*, 357-364.

Cox, C. (1926). *The early mental traits of three hundred geniuses*. Stanford, CA: Stanford University Press.

Cozens, F.W. (1927). Status of the problem of the relation of physical and mental ability. *American Physical Education Review, 32*, 127-155.

Craik, K.J.W. (1947). Theory of the human operator in control systems: I. The operator as an engineering system. *British Journal of Psychology, 38*, 56-61.

Craik, K.J.W. (1948). The theory of the human operator in control systems: II. Man as an element in a control system. *British Journal of Psychology, 38*, 142-148.

Crandall, V.C. (1963). Achievement. In H.W. Stevenson (Ed.), *Child psychology* (pp. 416-459). Chicago: University of Chicago Press.

Cratty, B.J. (1964). *Movement behavior and motor learning*. Philadelphia: Lea & Febiger.

Cratty, B.J. (1972). *Physical expressions of intelligence*. Englewood Cliffs, NJ: Prentice Hall.

Cropley, A.J. (1967). *Creativity*. London: Longmans, Green.

Crossman, J. (1977). *The effects of cognitive strategies on the performance of athletes*. Unpublished doctoral dissertation, Lakehead University, Thunder Bay, ON.

Davis, W.E., & Kelso, J.A.S. (1982). Analysis of "invariant characteristics" in the motor control of Down's syndrome and normal subjects. *Journal of Motor Behavior*, **14**, 194-212.

Day, W.F. (1969). On certain similarities between the philosophical investigations of Ludwig Wittgenstein and the operationism of B.F. Skinner. *Journal of the Experimental Analysis of Behavior*, **12**, 489-506.

Dayan, A. (1986). *Development of automatic and effortful processes in memory of movement location*. Unpublished doctoral dissertation, Louisiana State University, Baton Rouge.

Dayan, A., & Thomas, J.R. (in press). Intention to remember spatial locations in movement: Developmental considerations. *Human Performance*.

Deci, E.L. (1975). *Intrinsic motivation*. New York: Plenum Press.

DeMonbreun, B.G., & Mahoney, M.J. (1976). The effect of data return patterns on confidence in an hypothesis. In M.J. Mahoney (Ed.), *Scientist as subject: The psychological imperative* (pp. 181-186). Cambridge, MA: Ballinger.

Dewey, D., Brawley, L.R., & Allard, F. (1989). Do the TAIS attentional-style scales predict how visual information is processed? *Journal of Sport and Exercise Psychology*, **11**, 171-186.

Diamond, S.S., & Morton, D.R. (1978). Empirical landmarks in social psychology. *Personality and Social Psychology Bulletin*, **4**, 217-221.

Dickinson, J., & Goodman, D. (1986). Perspectives on motor learning theory and motor control. In L.D. Zaichkowsky & C.Z. Fuchs (Eds.), *The psychology of motor behavior: Development, control, learning and performance* (pp. 29-48). Ithaca, NY: Mouvement.

Dishman, R.K. (1982). Contemporary sport psychology. *Exercise and Sport Sciences Reviews*, **10**, 120-159.

Dishman, R.K. (1983). Identity crisis in North American sport psychology: Academics in professional issues. *Journal of Sport Psychology*, **5**, 123-134.

Dishman, R.K. (Ed.) (1988). *Exercise adherence: Its impact on public health*. Champaign, IL: Human Kinetics.

Dorfman, P.W. (1977). Timing and anticipation: A developmental perspective. *Journal of Motor Behavior*, **9**, 67-79.

Duda, J.L. (1989). Goal perspectives and behavior in sport and exercise settings. In C. Ames & M. Maehr (Eds.), *Advances in motivation and achievement—Vol. VI* (pp. 81-115). Greenwich, CT: JAI Press.

Duda, J.L. (1992). Motivation in sport settings: A goal perspective approach. In G.C. Roberts (Ed.), *Motivation in sport and exercise*. Champaign, IL: Human Kinetics.

Dunnett, M.D. (1966). Fads, fashions, and folderol in psychology. *American Psychologist*, **21**, 343-352.

Dweck, C.S. (1980). Learned helplessness in sport. In C.H. Nadeau, W.R. Halliwell, K.M. Newell, & G.C. Roberts (Eds.), *Psychology of motor behavior and sport—1979* (pp. 1-11). Champaign, IL: Human Kinetics.

Edwards, W.H. (1989). Contemporary and all-time notables. *Journal of Physical Education, Recreation and Dance*, **60**, 77-79.

Ellis, N.R. (1963). The stimulus trace and behavioral inadequacy. In N.R. Ellis (Ed.), *Handbook of mental deficiency*. New York: McGraw-Hill.

Ellis, N.R. (1970). Memory processes in retardates and normals. In N.R. Ellis (Ed.), *International review of research in mental retardation*. New York: Academic Press.

Ellis, J.D., Carron, A.V., & Bailey, D.A. (1975). Physical performance in boys 10 through 16 years. *Human Biology*, **47**, 263-281.

Elstein, A.S., Shulman, L.S., & Sprafka, S.A. (1978). *Medical problem solving: An analysis of clinical reasoning*. Cambridge, MA: Harvard University Press.

Engle, R.W., & Bukstel, L. (1978). Memory processes among bridge players of different expertise. *American Journal of Psychology*, **91**, 673-689.

Espenschade, A.S. (1940). Motor performance in adolescence including the study of relationships with measures of physical growth and maturity. *Monographs of the Society for Research in Child Development*, **5**, (1, Serial no. 24).

Ewing, M.E. (1981). *Achievement orientations and sport behavior of males and females*. Unpublished doctoral dissertation, University of Illinois, Urbana-Champaign.

Eysenck, H.J. (1966). Personality and experimental psychology. *Bulletin of the British Psychological Society*, **191**, 1-28.

Feldman, A.G. (1986). Once more on the equilibrium point hypothesis (model) for motor control. *Journal of Motor Behavior*, **18**, 17-54.

Feltz, D.L. (1987). Advancing knowledge in sport psychology: Strategies for expanding our conceptual frameworks. *Quest*, **39**, 243-254.

Feltz, D.L., & Landers, D.M. (1983). The effects of mental practice on motor skill learning and performance: A meta-analysis. *Journal of Sport Psychology*, **5**, 25-57.

Fentress, J.C. (1976). Dynamic boundaries of patterned behavior: Interaction and self-organization. In P.P.G. Bateson & R.A. Hinde (Eds.), *Growing points in ethology* (pp. 135-169). Cambridge, UK: Cambridge University Press.

Fishman, D.B., & Neigher, W.D. (1982). American psychology in the eighties: Who will buy? *American Psychologist*, **37**, 533-546.

Fitts, P.M. (1954). The information capacity of the human motor system in controlling the amplitude of movement. *Journal of Experimental Psychology*, **47**, 381-391.

Flavell, J.H. (1970). Developmental studies of mediated memory. In H.W. Reese & L.P. Lipsitt (Eds.), *Advances in child development and behavior* (Vol. 5). New York: Academic Press.

Ford, D. (1982). *The effects of cognitive strategies on swimming performance*. Unpublished master's thesis, Lakehead University, Thunder Bay, ON.

Forscher, B.K. (1963). Chaos in the brickyard. *Science*, **142**, 339.

Francis, R.J., & Rarick, G.L. (1959). Motor characteristics of the mentally retarded. *American Journal of Mental Deficiency*, **63**, 792-811.

Franks, C.M. (1979). *Annual review of behavior therapy* (Vol. 3). New York: Guilford Press.

French, K.E. (1985). *The relation of knowledge development to children's basketball performance*. Unpublished doctoral dissertation, Louisiana State University, Baton Rouge.

French, K.E., & Thomas, J.R. (1987). The relation of knowledge development to children's basketball performance. *Journal of Sport Psychology*, **9**, 15-32.

Frieze, I.H. (1976). Causal attributions and information seeking to explain success and failure. *Journal of Research in Personality*, **10**, 293-305.

Frostig, M., & Horne, D. (1964). *The Frostig program for the development of visual perception*. Chicago: Follett.

Gallagher, J.D. (1980). *Adult-child motor performance difference: A developmental perspective of control processing deficits*. Unpublished doctoral dissertation, Louisiana State University, Baton Rouge.

Gallagher, J.D. (1984). Influence of developmental information processing abilities on children's motor performance. In W.F. Straub & J.M. Williams (Eds.), *Cognitive sport psychology* (pp. 153-162). Lansing, NY: Sport Science Associates.

Gallagher, J.D., & Thomas, J.R. (1980). Effects of varying post-KR intervals upon children's motor performance. *Journal of Motor Behavior*, **12**, 41-46.

Gallagher, J.D., & Thomas, J.R. (1984). Rehearsal strategy effects on developmental differences for recall of a movement series. *Research Quarterly for Exercise and Sport*, **55**, 123-128.

Gallagher, J.D., & Thomas, J.R. (1986). Developmental effects of grouping and recoding on learning a movement series. *Research Quarterly for Exercise and Sport*, **57**, 117-127.

Gerson, R.F., & Thomas, J.R. (1977). Schema theory and practice variability within a neo-Piagetian framework. *Journal of Motor Behavior*, **9**, 127-134.

Gerson, R.F., & Thomas, J.R. (1978). A neo-Piagetian investigation of the serial position effect in children's motor learning. *Journal of Motor Behavior*, **10**, 95-104.

Gesell, A.L. (1946). The ontogenesis of infant behavior. In L. Carmichael (Ed.), *Manual of child psychology* (pp. 295-331). New York: Wiley.

Gesell, A.L., & Ilg, F.L. (1946). *The child from five to ten.* New York: Harper.

Gibbs, J.C. (1979). The meaning of ecologically oriented inquiry in contemporary psychology. *American Psychologist, 34,* 127-140.

Gibson, J.J. (1961). Ecological optics. *Vision Research, 1,* 253-262.

Gibson, J.J. (1966). *The senses considered as perceptual systems.* Boston: Houghton Mifflin.

Gibson, J.J. (1979). *The ecological approach to visual perception.* Boston: Houghton Mifflin.

Gill, D.L. (1981). Current research and future prospects in sport psychology. In G.A. Brooks (Ed.), *Perspectives on the academic discipline of physical education* (pp. 342-378). Champaign, IL: Human Kinetics.

Glass, G.V. (1977). Integrating findings: The meta-analysis of research. *Review of Research in Education, 5,* 351-379.

Glass, G.V., McGaw, B., & Smith, M. (1981). *Meta-analysis in social research.* Beverly Hills, CA: Sage.

Glassford, R.G. (1987). Methodological reconsiderations: The shifting paradigms. *Quest, 39,* 295-312.

Gleick, J. (1987). *Chaos: Making a new science.* New York: Penguin Books.

Gordon, I.E. (1989). *Theories of visual perception.* Chichester, UK: Wiley.

Gould, D., & Roberts, G.C. (1982). Modeling and motor skill acquisition. *Quest, 33,* 214-230.

Greene, P.H. (1972). Problems of organization of motor systems. In R. Rosen & F.M. Snell (Eds.), *Progress in theoretical biology* (Vol. 2). New York: Academic Press.

Greenwald, A.G. (1975). Consequences of prejudice against the null hypothesis. *Psychological Bulletin, 82,* 1-20.

Greenwald, A.G., Pratkanis, A.R., Leippe, M.R., & Baumgardner, M.H. (1986). Under what conditions does theory obstruct research progress? *Psychological Review, 93,* 216-229.

Griffin, N.S., & Keogh, J.F. (1982). A model for movement confidence. In J.A.S. Kelso & J.E. Clark (Eds.), *The development of movement control and coordination* (pp. 213-236). New York: Wiley.

Griffin, N.S., Keogh, J.F., & Maybee, R. (1984). Performer perceptions of movement confidence. *Journal of Sport Psychology, 6,* 395-407.

Griffith, C.R. (1926). *Psychology of coaching.* New York: Scribner's.

Griffith, C.R. (1928). *Psychology and athletics.* New York: Scribner's.

Gruber, H.E. (1989). Networks of enterprise in creative scientific work. In B. Gholson, W.R. Shadish, Jr., R.A. Neimeyer, & A.C. Houts (Eds.), *Psychology of science: Contributions to metascience* (pp. 246-265). Cambridge, UK: Cambridge University Press.

Haas, J., & Roberts, G.C. (1975). Effect of evaluative others upon learning and performance of a complex motor task. *Journal of Motor Behavior, 7,* 81-90.

Haken, H. (1983). *Synergetics—An introduction* (3rd ed.). Heidelberg, Germany: Springer-Verlag.

Haken, H. (1987). Information compression in biological systems. *Biological Cybernetics, 56*, 11-17.

Haken, H., Kelso, J.A.S., & Bunz, H. (1985). A theoretical model of phase transitions in human hand movements. *Biological Cybernetics, 51*, 347-357.

Hall, H. (1990). *A social-cognitive approach to goal setting: The mediating effects of achievement goals and perceived ability.* Unpublished doctoral dissertation, University of Illinois, Urbana-Champaign.

Halverson, H.M. (1931). An experimental study of prehension in infants by means of systematic cinema records. *Genetic Psychology Monographs, 10*, 107-286.

Hargens, L.L. (1978). Relations between work habits, research technologies, and eminence in science. *Sociology of Work and Occupations, 5*, 97-112.

Harris, D.V. (1987). Frontiers in psychology of exercise and sport. In M.J. Safrit & H.M. Eckert (Eds.), *The cutting edge in physical education and exercise science research* (pp. 42-52). Champaign, IL: Human Kinetics.

Harris, J.C., & Park, R.J. (1987). Guest editorial. *Quest, 39*, 227-230.

Harter, S. (1978). Effectance motivation reconsidered: Toward a developmental model. *Human Development, 21*, 34-64.

Hasher, L., & Zacks, R.T. (1979). Automatic and effortful processes in memory. *Journal of Experimental Psychology: General, 108*, 356-388.

Hatfield, B.D., & Landers, D.M. (1983). Psychophysiology—A new direction for sport psychology. *Journal of Sport Psychology, 5*, 243-259.

Hatfield, B.D., Landers, D.M., & Ray, W.J. (1987). Cardiovascular-CNS interactions in a highly trained, intentional attentive state: Elite marksmanship performance. *Psychophysiology, 24*, 542-549.

Hedges, L.V., & Olkin, I. (1985). *Statistical methods for meta-analysis.* New York: Academic Press.

Henderson, S.E., & Hall, D. (1982). Concomitants of clumsiness in young children. *Developmental Medicine and Child Neurology, 24*, 448-460.

Henry, F.M. (1948). Discrimination of the duration of a sound. *Journal of Experimental Psychology, 38*, 734-743.

Henry, F.M. (1953). Dynamic kinesthetic perception and adjustment. *Research Quarterly, 24*, 176-187.

Henry, F.M. (1958). Specificity vs. generality in learning motor skills. *Proceedings of the College of Physical Education Association, 61*, 126-128.

Henry, F.M. (1959). Reliability, measurement error, and intra-individual difference. *Research Quarterly, 30*, 21-24.

Henry, F.M. (1961). Stimulus complexity, movement complexity, age and sex in relation to reaction latency and speed of limb movements. *Research Quarterly, 32*, 353-366.

Henry, F.M. (1964). Physical education—An academic discipline. *Proceedings of the College of Physical Education Association, 67*, 6-9.

Henry, F.M. (1974). Variable and constant performance errors within a group of individuals. *Journal of Motor Behavior, 6*, 149-154.

Henry, F.M. (1975). Absolute error versus "E" in target accuracy. *Journal of Motor Behavior, 7*, 227-228.

Henry, F.M. (1978). The academic discipline of physical education. *Quest, 29*, 13-29.

Henry, F.M. (1981a). The evolution of the memory drum theory of neuromotor reaction. In G.A. Brooks (Ed.), *Perspectives on the academic discipline of physical education* (pp. 301-322). Champaign, IL: Human Kinetics.

Henry, F.M. (1981b). Stability-instability of the motor memory trace: A modification of the 1960 memory drum theory. In G.C. Roberts & D.M. Landers (Eds.), *Psychology of motor behavior and sport—1980* (pp. 60-70). Champaign, IL: Human Kinetics.

Henry, F.M. (1986). Development of the motor memory trace and control program. *Journal of Motor Behavior, 18*, 77-100.

Henry, F.M., & DeMoor, J.C. (1956). Lactic and alactic oxygen consumption in moderate exercise of graded intensity. *Journal of Applied Physiology, 8*, 608-614.

Henry, F.M., & Rogers, D.E. (1960). Increased response latency for complicated movements and a memory drum theory of neuromotor reaction. *Research Quarterly, 31*, 448-458.

Henry, F.M., & Trafton, I.R. (1951). The velocity curve of sprint running with some observations on the muscle viscosity factor. *Research Quarterly, 22*, 409-422.

Highmore, G., & Taylor, W.R. (1954). A factorial analysis of athletic ability. *The British Journal of Statistical Psychology, 7*, 1-8.

Hill, A.V. (1927). *Muscular movement in man.* New York: McGraw-Hill.

Hubert, J.Z. (1978). Creativity: A definition based on the concept of negentropy. *Dialectics and Humanism, 2.*

Hudson, L. (1972). *The cult of the fact.* London: Cape.

Hull, C.L. (1943). *Principles of behavior.* New York: Appleton-Century-Crofts.

Humphries, C.A. (1986). *Skill and knowledge base attributes of young baseball players.* Unpublished doctoral dissertation, Louisiana State University, Baton Rouge.

Hunter, I.M.L. (1968). Mental calculation. In P.C. Wason & P.N. Johnson-Laird (Eds.), *Thinking and reasoning* (pp. 341-351). Baltimore: Penguin.

Hyman, R. (1953). Stimulus information as a determinant of reaction time. *Journal of Experimental Psychology, 45*, 188-196.

Ismail, A.H., Kane, J.E., & Kirkendall, D.R. (1969). Relationships among intellectual and non-intellectual variables. *Research Quarterly, 40*, 83-92.

James, W. (1890). *The principles of psychology* (Vol. 1). New York: Holt.

Jansen, B.J., & Whiting, H.T.A. (1984). Sheldon's physical-psychical topology revisited. *Journal of Research in Personality, 18,* 432-441.

Jenkins, J.J. (1974). Remember that old theory of memory? Well, forget it! *American Psychologist, 29,* 785-795.

Johnson, W.R. (1949). A study of emotion revealed in two types of athletic sports contests. *Research Quarterly, 20,* 72-79.

Johnson, W.R., & Hutton, D.H. (1955). Effects of a combative sport upon personality dynamics as measured by a projective test. *Research Quarterly, 26,* 49-53.

Jones, B. (1974). Role of central monitoring of efference in short term memory for movements. *Journal of Experimental Psychology, 102,* 37-43.

Jones, E.R. (1988, Winter). Philosophical tension in a scientific discipline: So what else is new? *NASPSPA Newsletter, 14*(1), 10-16.

Jones, H.E. (1949). *Motor performance and growth.* Berkeley: University of California Press.

Jordan, N. (1968). *Themes in speculative psychology.* Tavistock, UK: Tavistock.

Kaiser, H.F., Hunda, S., & Bianchini, J.D. (1971). Relating factors between studies based on different individuals. *Multivariate Behavioral Research, 6,* 409-422.

Kantor, J.R. (1966). Feelings and emotions as scientific events. *Psychological Record, 16,* 377-404.

Keele, S.W. (1968). Movement control in skilled motor performance. *Psychological Bulletin, 70,* 387-403.

Kelso, J.A.S. (1975). Planning, efferent, and receptor components in movement coding (Doctoral dissertation, University of Wisconsin, 1975). *University of Oregon: Microform Publication,* **BF371,** 153-173.

Kelso, J.A.S. (1977a). Motor control mechanisms underlying human movement reproduction. *Journal of Experimental Psychology: Human Perception and Performance, 3,* 529-543.

Kelso, J.A.S. (1977b). Planning and efferent commands in the coding of movement. *Journal of Motor Behavior, 9,* 33-47.

Kelso, J.A.S. (1981). On the oscillatory basis of movement. *Bulletin of the Psychonomic Society, 18,* 63.

Kelso, J.A.S. (Ed.) (1982a). *Human motor behavior: An introduction.* Hillsdale, NJ: Erlbaum.

Kelso, J.A.S. (1982b). The process approach to understanding human motor behavior: An introduction. In J.A.S. Kelso (Ed.), *Human motor behavior: An introduction* (pp. 3-19). Hillsdale, NJ: Erlbaum.

Kelso, J.A.S. (1984). Phase transitions and critical behavior in human bimanual coordination. *American Journal of Physiology: Regulatory, Integrative and Comparative, 15,* R1000-R1004.

Kelso, J.A.S. (1986). Pattern formation in multi-degree of freedom speech and limb movements. *Experimental Brain Research Supplement, 15,* 105-128.

Kelso, J.A.S., & Clark, J.E. (Eds.) (1982). *The development of movement control and co-ordination*. New York: Wiley.

Kelso, J.A.S., Cook, E., Olson, M.E., & Epstein, W. (1975). Allocation of attention and the locus of adaptation to displaced vision. *Journal of Experimental Psychology: Human Perception and Performance, 1*, 237-245.

Kelso, J.A.S., Goodman, D., Stamm, C.L., & Hayes, C. (1979). Movement coding and memory in retarded children. *American Journal of Mental Deficiency, 83*, 601-611.

Kelso, J.A.S., Holt, K.G., Kugler, P.N., & Turvey, M.T. (1980). On the concept of coordinative structures as dissipative structures: II. Empirical lines of convergence. In G.E. Stelmach & J. Requin (Eds.), *Tutorials in motor behavior* (pp. 49-70). Amsterdam: North-Holland.

Kelso, J.A.S., Holt, K.G., Rubin, P., & Kugler, P.N. (1981). Patterns of human interlimb coordination emerge from the properties of nonlinear, limit-cycle oscillatory processes: Theory and data. *Journal of Motor Behavior, 13*, 226-261.

Kelso, J.A.S., & Kay, B.A. (1987). Information and control: A macroscopic analysis of perception-action coupling. In H. Heuer & A.F. Sanders (Eds.), *Perspectives on perception and action* (pp. 3-32). Hillsdale, NJ: Erlbaum.

Kelso, J.A.S., Saltzman, E., & Tuller, B. (1986). The dynamical perspective on speech production: Data and theory. *Journal of Phonetics, 14*, 29-59.

Kelso, J.A.S., & Scholz, J.P. (1985). Co-operative phenomena in biological motion. In H. Haken (Ed.), *Complex systems: Operational approaches in neurobiology, physical systems and computers* (pp. 124-149). Berlin: Springer-Verlag.

Kelso, J.A.S., Scholz, J.P., & Schöner, G. (1986). Nonequilibrium phase transitions in coordinated biological motion: Critical fluctuations. *Physics Letters A, 118*, 279-284.

Kelso, J.A.S., & Schöner, G. (1987). Toward a physical/synergetic theory of biological coordination. In R. Graham & A. Wunderlin (Eds.), *Lasers and synergetics* (pp. 224-237). Berlin-Heidelberg: Springer.

Kelso, J.A.S., & Schöner, G. (1988). Self-organization of coordinative movement patterns. *Human Movement Science, 7*, 27-46.

Kelso, J.A.S., Schöner, G., Scholz, J.P., & Haken, H. (1987). Phase-locked modes, phase transitions and component oscillators in biological motion. *Physica Scripta, 35*, 79-87.

Kelso, J.A.S., Southard, D.L., & Goodman, D. (1979). On the nature of human interlimb coordination. *Science, 203*, 1029-1031.

Kelso, J.A.S., Stelmach, G.E., & Wanamaker, W.M. (1974). Behavioral and neurological parameters of the nerve compression block. *Journal of Motor Behavior, 6*, 179-190.

Kelso, J.A.S., Stelmach, G.E., & Wanamaker, W.M. (1976). The continuing saga of nerve compression block. *Journal of Motor Behavior*, **8**, 155-160.

Kelso, J.A.S., & Tuller, B. (1984). Converging evidence in support of common dynamical principles for speech and movement coordination. *American Journal of Physiology*, **246**, R928-R935.

Kelso, J.A.S., Wallace, S.A., Stelmach, G.E., & Weitz, G.A. (1975). Sensory and motor impairment in the nerve compression block. *Quarterly Journal of Experimental Psychology*, **27**, 123-129.

Kendler, H.H. (1981). *Psychology: A science in conflict*. New York: Oxford University Press.

Keogh, J.F. (1965). *Motor performance of elementary school children*. Unpublished technical report, University of California, Department of Physical Education, Los Angeles.

Keogh, J.F. (1968). *Developmental evaluation of limb movement tasks*. Unpublished technical report, University of California, Department of Physical Education, Los Angeles.

Keogh, J.F. (1969). *Change in motor performance during early school years*. Unpublished technical report, University of California, Department of Physical Education, Los Angeles.

Keogh, J.F. (1971). Motor control as a unifying concept in the study of motor development. *Motor development symposium*. Berkeley: University of California.

Keogh, J.F. (1977). Study of motor development. *Quest*, **28**, 76-88.

Keogh, J.F. (1978). Movement outcomes as conceptual guidelines in the perceptual-motor maze. *Journal of Special Education*, **12**, 321-330.

Keogh, J.F. (1981). A movement development framework and a perceptual-cognitive perspective. In G.A. Brooks (Ed.), *Perspectives on the academic discipline of physical education* (pp. 211-233). Champaign, IL: Human Kinetics.

Keogh, J.F. (1982). The study of movement learning disabilities. In J.P. Das, R.F. Mulcahy, & A.E. Wall (Eds.), *Theory and research in learning disabilities* (pp. 237-251). New York: Plenum Press.

Keogh, J.F., Griffin, N.S., & Spector, R. (1981). Observer perceptions of movement confidence. *Research Quarterly for Exercise and Sport*, **52**, 465-473.

Keogh, J.F., & Sugden, D.A. (1985). *Movement skill development*. New York: Macmillan.

Keogh, J.F., Sugden, D.A., Reynard, C.L., & Calkins, J.A. (1979). Identification of clumsy children: Comparisons and comments. *Journal of Human Movement Studies*, **5**, 32-41.

Kephart, N.C. (1960). *The slow learner in the classroom*. Columbus, OH: Merrill.

Koch, S. (1969). Psychology cannot be a coherent science. *Psychology Today*, **3**, 14.

Koestler, A. (1964). *The act of creation*. New York: Macmillan.

Krawiec, T.S. (Ed.) (1974). *The psychologists* (Vol. 2). New York: Oxford University Press.

Kroll, W.P. (1971). *Perspectives in physical education*. New York: Academic Press.

Kroll, W., & Lewis, G. (1970). America's first sport psychologist. *Quest*, **13**, 1-4.

Kugler, P.N. (1986). A morphological perspective on the origin and evolution of movement patterns. In M.G. Wade & H.T.A. Whiting (Eds.), *Motor development in children: Aspects of coordination and control* (pp. 459-525). Dordrecht, Netherlands: Martinus Nijhoff.

Kugler, P.N., Kelso, J.A.S., & Turvey, M.T. (1980). On the concept of coordinative structures as dissipative structures: I. Theoretical lines of convergence. In G.E. Stelmach & J. Requin (Eds.), *Tutorials in motor behavior* (pp. 3-47). Amsterdam: North-Holland.

Kugler, P.N., Kelso, J.A.S., & Turvey, M.T. (1982). On coordination and control in naturally developing systems. In J.A.S. Kelso & J.E. Clark (Eds.), *The development of movement control and coordination* (pp. 5-78). New York: Wiley.

Kugler, P.N., & Turvey, M.T. (1987). *Information, natural law and the self-assembly of rhythmic movement*. Hillsdale, NJ: Erlbaum.

Kuhn, T.S. (1962). *The structure of scientific revolutions*. Chicago: University of Chicago Press.

Kuhn, T.S. (1970). Reflections on my critics. In I. Lakatos & A. Musgrave (Eds.), *Criticism and the growth of knowledge* (pp. 231-278). Cambridge, UK: Cambridge University Press.

Kuhn, T.S. (1973). Second thoughts on paradigms. In F. Suppe (Ed.), *The structure of scientific theories* (pp. 459-482). Urbana: University of Illinois Press.

Kuhn, T.S. (1977). *The essential tension: Selected studies in scientific tradition and change*. Chicago: Chicago University Press.

Laabs, G.T. (1973). Retention characteristics of different reproduction cues in motor short-term memory. *Journal of Experimental Psychology*, **100**, 168-177.

Lachman, S.J. (1960). *The foundations of science*. New York: Vantage Press.

Lakatos, I. (1970a). Falsification and the methodology of scientific research programmes. In I. Lakatos & A. Musgrave (Eds.), *Criticism and the growth of knowledge* (pp. 91-196). Cambridge, UK: Cambridge University Press.

Lakatos, I. (1970b). History of science and its rational reconstruction. In R.C. Buck & R.S. Cohen (Eds.), *Boston studies in the philosophy of science* (Vol. 8). Dordrect, Netherlands: Reidel.

Lakatos, I., & Musgrave, A. (Eds.) (1970). *Criticism and the growth of knowledge*. Cambridge, UK: Cambridge University Press.

Lakatos, I., & Zahar, E. (1975). Why did Copernicus's programme supersede Ptolemy's? In R. Westman (Ed.),*The Copernican achievement*. Berkeley, CA: University of California Press.

Landauer, R. (1981). Nonlinearity, multistability and fluctuations. *American Journal of Physiology*, **241**, R107-R113.

Landers, D.M. (1983). Whatever happened to theory testing in sport psychology? *Journal of Sport Psychology*, **5**, 135-158.

Landers, D.M., Boutcher, S.H., & Wang, M.Q. (1986a). The history and status of the *Journal of Sport Psychology*: 1979-1985. *Journal of Sport Psychology*, **8**, 149-163.

Landers, D.M., Boutcher, S.H., & Wang, M.Q. (1986b). A psychobiological study of archery performance. *Research Quarterly for Exercise and Sport*, **57**, 236-244.

Langley, P.W., Simon, H.A., Bradshaw, G., & Zytkow, J. (1987). *Scientific discovery: Computational explorations of the creative process.* Cambridge, MA: MIT Press.

Larkin, J., McDermott, J., Simon, D.P., & Simon, H.A. (1980). Expert and novice performance in solving physics problems. *Science*, **208**, 1335-1342.

Laszlo, J.I., & Bairstow, P.J. (1985). *Perceptual-motor behaviour: Developmental assessment and therapy.* London: Holt, Rinehart & Winston.

Lawther, J.D. (1951). *The psychology of coaching.* Englewood Cliffs, NJ: Prentice Hall.

Leavitt, J.L., & Carron, A.V. (1969). Intra-task reliability and specificity of individual differences in reminiscence in two motor learning tasks. *Journal of Motor Behavior*, **1**, 275-284.

Leonard, F.E., & Afflect, G.B. (1947). *A guide to the history of physical education.* Philadelphia: Lea & Febiger.

LeUnes, A., Wolf, P., Ripper, N., & Anding, K. (1990). Classic references in *Journal of Sport Psychology*, 1979-1987. *Journal of Exercise and Sport Psychology*, **12**, 74-81.

Levey, A.B., & Martin, I. (1988). Empiricism, theory, and science. *Journal of Psychophysiology*, **2**, 3-4.

Loy, J.W. (1974). A brief history of the North American Society for the Psychology of Sport and Physical Activity. In M.G. Wade & R. Martens (Eds.), *Psychology of motor behavior and sport—1973.* Champaign, IL: Human Kinetics.

Lichtenstein, P.E. (1971). A behavioral approach to "phenomenological data." *Psychological Record*, **21**, 1-16.

Mach, E. (1896). On the part played by accident in invention and discovery. *Monist*, **6**, 161-175.

Maehr, M.L., & Nicholls, J.G. (1980). Culture and achievement motivation: A second look. In N. Warren (Ed.), *Studies in cross-cultural psychology* (pp. 221-267). New York: Academic Press.

Magill, R.A. (1990). Motor learning is meaningful for physical educators. *Quest*, **42**, 126-133.

Mahoney, M.J. (1976). *Scientist as subject: The psychological imperative.* Cambridge, MA: Ballinger.

Malina, R.M. (1979). Secular changes in growth, maturation, and physical performance. *Exercise and Sport Sciences Reviews*, **6**, 203-255.

Malina, R.M. (1981). Growth, maturation, and human performance. In G.A. Brooks (Ed.), *Perspectives on the academic discipline of physical education* (pp. 190-210). Champaign, IL: Human Kinetics.

Martens, R. (1977). *Sport competition anxiety test*. Champaign, IL: Human Kinetics.

Martens, R. (1979). About smocks and jocks. *Journal of Sport Psychology*, **1**, 94-99.

Martens, R. (1980). From smocks to jocks: A new adventure for sport psychologists. In P. Klavora & J.V. Daniel (Eds.), *Psychological and sociological factors in sport* (pp. 55-62). Toronto: University of Toronto.

Martens, R. (1987). Science, knowledge, and sport psychology. *The Sport Psychologist*, **1**, 29-55.

McCain, G., & Segal, E.M. (1969). *The game of science* (2nd ed.). Monterey, CA: Brooks/Cole.

McCall, R.B. (1977). Challenges to a science of developmental psychology. *Child Development*, **48**, 333-344.

McCaskill, C.L., & Wellman, B.L. (1938). A study of common motor achievements at the preschool ages. *Child Development*, **9**, 141-150.

McClelland, D.C. (1951). *Personality*. New York: Dryden.

McClelland, D.C. (1961). *The achieving society*. Princeton, NJ: Van Nostrand.

McClelland, D.C. (1963). The calculated risk: An aspect of scientific performance. In C.W. Taylor & F. Barron (Eds.), *Scientific creativity* (pp. 184-192). New York: Wiley.

McCloy, C.H. (1930). Character building through physical education. *Research Quarterly*, **1**, 41-61.

McCloy, C.H. (1934). The measurement of general motor capacity and general motor ability. *Research Quarterly*, **5**(Suppl. 5), 45-61.

McGuire, W.J. (1973). The yin and yang of social psychology: Seven Koan. *Journal of Personality and Social Psychology*, **26**, 446-456.

McKeithen, K.B., Reitman, J.S., Rueter, H.H., & Hirtle, S.C. (1981). Knowledge organization and skill differences in computer programmers. *Cognitive Psychology*, **13**, 307-325.

McKenzie, T.L., & Rushall, B.S. (1974). Effects of self-recording contingencies on improving attendance and performance in a competitive swimming training environment. *Journal of Applied Behavior Analysis*, **7**, 199-206.

McKinnon, E. (1985). *The effects of cognitive strategies on the ergometer performance of female rowers*. Unpublished master's thesis, Lakehead University, Thunder Bay, ON.

McNair, D.M., Lorr, M., & Droppleman, L.F. (1971). *Profile of Mood States manual*. San Diego: Educational and Industrial Testing Service.

McPherson, S.L. (1987). *The development of children's expertise in tennis: Knowledge structure and sport performance*. Unpublished doctoral dissertation, Louisiana State University, Baton Rouge.

McPherson, S.L., & Thomas, J.R. (1989). Relation of knowledge and precision in boys' tennis: Age and expertise. *Journal of Experimental Child Psychology*, **48**, 190-211.

Meichenbaum, D.H. (1977). *Cognitive-Behavior Modification: An Integrative Approach*. New York: Plenum.

Meijer, O.G., & Roth, K. (Eds.) (1988). *Complex movement behaviour: 'The' motor-action controversy*. Amsterdam: North-Holland.

Melton, A.W. (1947). *Apparatus tests*. Washington, DC: U.S. Government Printing Office.

Meltzoff, A.N., & Moore, M.K. (1985). Cognitive foundations and social functions of imitation and intermodal representation in infancy. In J. Mehler & R. Fox (Eds.), *Neonate cognition: Beyond the blooming, buzzing confusion*. Hillsdale, NJ: Erlbaum.

Miles, W.R. (1931). Studies in physical exertion: II. Individual and group reaction time in football charging. *Research Quarterly*, **2**, 5-13.

Miller, G.A. (1956). The magical number seven, plus or minus two: Some limits on our capacity for processing information. *Psychological Review*, **63**, 81-97.

Miller, J. (1982). Discrete versus continuous stage models of human information processing: In search of partial output. *Journal of Experimental Psychology: Human Perception and Performance*, **8**, 273-296.

Miller, J. (1983). Can response preparation begin before stimulus-recognition finishes? *Journal of Experimental Psychology: Human Perception and Performance*, **9**, 161-182.

Mitchell, B.F. (1977). *Children's motor responses to precision KR: A neo-Piagetian interpretation*. Unpublished doctoral dissertation, Florida State University, Tallahassee.

Mitroff, I.I. (1974a). Norms and counter-norms in a select group of the Apollo moon scientists: A case study of the ambivalence of scientists. *American Sociological Review*, **39**, 579-595.

Mitroff, I.I. (1974b). *The subjective side of science*. New York: Elsevier Science.

Moon, D.H. (1975). *Developmental variables in children's performance rhythm ability*. Unpublished doctoral dissertation, Florida State University, Tallahassee.

Morford, W.R. (1966). The value of supplementary visual information during practice on dynamic kinesthetic learning. *Research Quarterly*, **37**, 393-405.

Morgan, W.P. (1980). Sport personology: The credulous-skeptical argument in perspective. In W.F. Straub (Ed.), *Sport psychology: An analysis of athlete behavior* (2nd ed.) (pp. 330-339). Ithaca, NY: Mouvement.

Morris, P.R., & Whiting, H.T.A. (1971). *Motor impairment and compensatory education*. London: Bell.

Murphy, G.L., & Wright, J.C. (1984). Changes in conceptual structure with expertise: Differences between real-world experts and novices.

Journal of Experimental Psychology: Learning, Memory and Cognition, **10**, 144-155.

Neisser, U. (1976). *Cognition and reality: Principles and implications of cognitive psychology.* San Francisco: Freeman.

Neisser, U. (1979). The control of information pick-up in selective looking. In A.D. Pick (Ed.), *Perception and its development: A tribute to Eleanor Gibson.* Hillsdale, NJ: Erlbaum.

Nelson, J.K., Thomas, J.R., Nelson, K.R., & Abraham, P.C. (1986). Gender differences in children's throwing performance: Biology and environment. *Research Quarterly for Exercise and Sport,* **57**, 280-287.

Nelson, K.R., Thomas, J.R., & Nelson, J.K. (1991). Longitudinal changes in throwing performances: Gender differences. *Research Quarterly for Exercise and Sport,* **62**, 105-108.

Newell, K.M. (1985). Motor skill acquisition and mental retardation: Overview of traditional and current orientations. In J.E. Clark & J.H. Humphrey (Eds.), *Motor development: Current selected research* (Vol. 1). Princeton, NJ: Princeton Press.

Newell, K.M. (1987). On masters and apprentices in physical education. *Quest,* **39**, 88-96.

Newell, K.M., & Barclay, C.R. (1982). Developing knowledge about action. In J.A.S. Kelso & J.E. Clark (Eds.), *The development of movement control and coordination* (pp. 175-212). Chichester, UK: Wiley.

Nicholls, J.G. (1984). Achievement motivation: Conceptions of ability, subjective experience, task choice, and performance. *Psychological Review,* **91**, 328-346.

Nicholls, J.G. (1989). *The competitive ethos and democratic education.* Cambridge, MA: Harvard University Press.

Nicholls, J.G. (1992). The general and the specific in the development and expression of achievement motivation. In G.C. Roberts (Ed.), *Motivation in sport and exercise.* Champaign, IL: Human Kinetics.

Nideffer, R.M. (1976a). *The inner athlete.* San Diego, CA: Enhanced Performance Systems.

Nideffer, R.M. (1976b). The test of attentional and interpersonal style. *Journal of Personality and Social Psychology,* **34**, 394-404.

Nideffer, R.M. (1981). *The ethics and practice of applied sport psychology.* Ithaca, NY: Mouvement.

Nideffer, R.M. (1983). The injured athlete: Psychological factors in treatment. *Orthopedic Clinics of North America,* **14**(2), 373-385.

Nideffer, R.M. (1987a). Psychological preparation of the highly competitive athlete. *The Physician and Sportsmedicine,* **18**(10), 85-92.

Nideffer, R.M. (1987b). Theoretical and practical relationships between attention, anxiety, and performance in sports. In D. Hackfort & C. Spielberger (Eds.), *Anxiety in sports: An international perspective.* New York: Hemisphere.

Nideffer, R.M., & Sharpe, R. (1978). *A.C.T.: Attention Control Training*. New York: Wynden Books.

Nisbett, R.E., & Wilson, T.D. (1977). Telling more than we can know: Verbal reports on mental processes. *Psychological Review*, **84**, 231-259.

Norman, D.A. (1968). Toward a theory of memory and attention. *Psychological Review*, **75**, 522-536.

Norman, D.A. (1969). *Memory and attention*. New York: Wiley.

Norman, D.A., & Shallice, T. (1985). Attention to action: Willed and automatic control of behavior. In R.J. Davidson, G.E. Schwartz, & D. Shapiro (Eds.), *Consciousness and self-regulation: Advances in Research* (Vol. IV). New York: Plenum Press.

Norrie, M.L. (1967). Practice effects on reaction latency for simple and complex movements. *Research Quarterly*, **38**, 79-85.

Nunley, R.L. (1965). A physical fitness program for the mentally retarded in the public schools. *Physical Therapy*, **45**, 949-954.

Oliver, J.N. (1958). The effect of physical conditioning exercises and activities on the mental characteristics of educationally sub-normal boys. *British Journal of Educational Psychology*, **28**, 155-165.

O'Neal, F.W. (1936). A behavior frequency rating scale for the measurement of character personality in high school physical education classes for boys. *Research Quarterly*, **7**, 67-76.

Ornstein, P.A. (Ed.) (1978). *Memory development in children*. Hillsdale, NY: Erlbaum.

Park, R.J. (1981). The emergence of the academic discipline of physical education in the United States. In G.A. Brooks (Ed.), *Perspectives on the academic discipline of physical education* (pp. 20-45). Champaign, IL: Human Kinetics.

Pascual-Leone, J., & Smith, J. (1969). The encoding and decoding of symbols by children: A new experimental paradigm and neo-Piagetian model. *Journal of Experimental Child Psychology*, **8**, 328-355.

Pattee, H. (1976). Physical theories of biological coordination. In M. Grene and E. Mendelsohn (Eds.), *Boston Studies in the Philosophy of Science* (pp. 153-173). Boston: Reidel.

Piaget, J. (1952). *The origins of intelligence*. New York: International Universities Press.

Pierce, C.G. (1977). *Observational learning: Temporal spacing and retention of a model presentation of a gross motor skill*. Unpublished master's thesis, Florida State University, Tallahassee.

Planck, M. (1949). *Scientific autobiography and other papers* (F. Gaynor, Trans.). New York: Philosophical Library.

Platt, J.R. (1964, October). Strong inference. *Science*, **146**, 347-352.

Polanyi, M. (1958). *Personal knowledge*. London: Routledge & Kegan Paul.

Polanyi, M. (1967). *The tacit dimension*. London: Routledge & Kegan Paul.

Pole, D. (1958). *The late philosophy of Wittgenstein*. London: Athlone Press.

Popper, K. (1972). *The logic of scientific discovery*. London: Hutchinson.

Quine, W.V., & Ullian, J.S. (1970). *The web of belief*. New York: Random House.

Rarick, G.L. (1937). An analysis of the speed factor in simple athletic activities. *Research Quarterly*, **8**, 89-105.

Rarick, G.L. (1961). *Motor development during infancy and childhood* (2nd ed.). Madison, WI: College Printing.

Rarick, G.L. (1967). The domain of physical education. *Quest*, **9**, 49-52.

Rarick, G.L. (Ed.) (1973). *Physical activity: Human growth and development*. New York: Academic Press.

Rarick, G.L. (1980). The factor structure of the motor domain of mentally retarded children and adolescents. In M. Ostyn, G. Beunen, & J. Simons (Eds.), *Kinanthropometry II* (pp. 149-160). Baltimore: University Park Press.

Rarick, G.L. (1982). Descriptive research and process-oriented explanations of the motor development of children. In J.A.S. Kelso & J.E. Clark (Eds.), *The development of movement control and co-ordination* (pp. 275-291). Chichester, UK: Wiley.

Rarick, G.L., Dobbins, D.A., & Broadhead, G.D. (1976). *The motor domain and its correlates in educationally handicapped children*. Englewood Cliffs, NJ: Prentice Hall.

Rarick, G.L., & Oyster, N. (1964). Physical maturity, muscular strength, and motor performance of young school-aged boys. *Research Quarterly*, **35**, 523-531.

Rarick, G.L., Rapaport, I.F., & Seefeldt, V. (1964). Bone development in Down's Disease. *American Journal of Diseases of Children*, **107**, 7-13.

Rarick, G.L., Rapaport, I.F., & Seefeldt, V. (1965). Age of appearance of ossification centres of the hand and wrist in children with Down's Disease. *Journal of Mental Deficiency Research*, **9**, 24-30.

Rarick, G.L., Rapaport, I.F., & Seefeldt, V. (1966). Long bone growth in Down's Syndrome. *American Journal of Diseases of Children*, **112**, 566-571.

Rarick, G.L., & Smoll, F.L. (1967). Stability of growth in strength and motor performance from childhood to adolescence. *Human Biology*, **39**, 295-306.

Rarick, G.L., & Thompson, J.A.J. (1956). Roentgenographic measures of leg muscle size and ankle extensor strength of seven-year-old children. *Research Quarterly*, **27**, 321-332.

Rarick, G.L., Wainer, H., Thissen, D., & Seefeldt, V. (1975). A double logistic comparison of growth patterns of normal children and children with Down's Syndrome. *Annals of Human Biology*, **2**, 339-346.

Rarick, G.L., Widdop, J.H., & Broadhead, G.D. (1970). The physical fitness and motor performance of educable mentally retarded children. *Exceptional Children*, **36**, 509-519.

Reed, E.S. (1982). An outline of a theory of action systems. *Journal of Motor Behavior*, **14**, 98-134.

Reed, E.S. (1988). Applying the theory of action systems to the study of motor skills. In O.G. Meijer & K. Roth (Eds.), *Complex motor behaviour: 'The' motor-action controversy* (pp. 45-86). Amsterdam: North-Holland.

Reichenbach, H. (1938). *Experience and prediction.* Chicago: University of Chicago Press.

Reid, G. (1980). Overt and covert rehearsal in short-term motor memory of mentally retarded and nonretarded persons. *American Journal of Mental Deficiency*, **85**, 69-77.

Renshaw, P. (1975). The nature and study of human movement: A philosophical examination. *Journal of Human Movement Studies*, **1**, 5-11.

Rice, Scott. (1984). *It Was a Dark and Stormy Night: The Best (?) From the Bulwer-Lytton Contest.* New York: Viking.

Richter, C.P. (1953). Free research versus design research. *Science*, **118**, 91-93.

Ricoeur, P. (1966). *Freedom and nature: The voluntary and the involuntary.* Evanston, IL: Northwestern University Press.

Roberton, M.A. (1978). Longitudinal evidence for developmental stages in the forceful overarm throw. *Journal of Human Movement Studies*, **4**, 167-175.

Roberton, M.A. (1982). Describing 'stages' within and across motor tasks. In J.A.S. Kelso & J.E. Clark (Eds.), *The development of movement control and co-ordination* (pp. 293-307). Chichester, UK: Wiley.

Roberton, M.A. (1986). Developmental changes in the relative timing of locomotion. In H.T.A. Whiting & M.G. Wade (Eds.), *Themes in motor development* (pp. 279-293). Dordrecht, Netherlands: Martinus Nijhoff.

Roberts, G.C. (1969). *Effect of presence of others, cooperative and competitive, on risk taking and performance.* Unpublished doctoral dissertation, University of Illinois, Urbana-Champaign.

Roberts, G.C. (1971). *Risk taking behavior in sport and physical education.* Invited presentation to the Faculty of Physical Education and Recreation of the State University College at Brockport, NY.

Roberts, G.C. (1973). The rise of European nationalism: Some possible implications for the pattern of physical education and sport. In E.F. Zeigler (Ed.), *A history of sport and physical education to 1900* (pp. 309-317). Champaign, IL: Human Kinetics.

Roberts, G.C. (1975). Win-loss causal attributions of Little League players. *Mouvement*, **7**, 315-322.

Roberts, G.C. (1978). Children's assignment of responsibility for winning and losing. In F.L. Smoll & R.E. Smith (Eds.), *Psychological perspectives on youth sports* (pp. 145-172). Washington, DC: Hemisphere.

Roberts, G.C. (1982). Achievement motivation in sport. In R. Terjung (Ed.), *Exercise and Sport Science Reviews* (Vol. 10) (pp. 236-269). Philadelphia: Franklin Institute Press.

Roberts, G.C. (1984). Achievement motivation in children's sport. In J.G. Nicholls (Ed.), *The development of achievement motivation* (pp. 251-281). Greenwich, CT: JAI Press.

Roberts, G.C. (1985). Graduate education in an age of change. *The Physical Educator*, **43**, 106-108, 160-161.

Roberts, G.C. (1989). When motivation matters: The need to expand the conceptual model. In J.S. Skinner, C.B. Corbin, D.M. Landers, P.E. Martin, & C.L. Wells (Eds.), *Future directions in exercise and sport science research* (pp. 77-84). Champaign, IL: Human Kinetics.

Roberts, G.C. (1991). Graduate education in kinesiology: A cross-disciplinary approach. In R. Park & H. Eckert (Eds.), *The Academy papers: New possibilities, new paradigms?* Champaign, IL: Human Kinetics.

Roberts, G.C. (1992). Motivation in sport and exercise: Conceptual constraints and conceptual convergence. In G.C. Roberts (Ed.), *Motivation in sport and exercise*. Champaign, IL: Human Kinetics.

Roberts, G.C., & Kimiecik, J. (1989). Sport psychology in East Germany: An interview with Gerd Konzag. *The Sport Psychologist*, **3**, 72-77.

Roberts, G.C., Kleiber, D.A., & Duda, J.L. (1981). An analysis of motivation in children's sport: The role of perceived competence in participation. *Journal of Sport Psychology*, **3**, 206-216.

Roberts, G.C., & Pascuzzi, D. (1979). Causal attributions in sport: Some theoretical implications. *Journal of Sport Psychology*, **1**, 203-211.

Roe, A. (1952a). *The making of a scientist*. New York: Dodd, Mead.

Roe, A. (1952b). A psychologist examines 64 eminent scientists. *Scientific American*, **187**(5), 21-25.

Rosen, R. (Ed.) (1985). *Theoretical biology and complexity*. New York: Academic Press.

Rudisill, M.E., & Singer, R.N. (1988). Influence of causal dimension orientation on persistence, performance and expectations of performance during perceived failure. *Journal of Human Movement Studies*, **15**, 215-228.

Rushall, B.S. (1960). *An elementary study of factors affecting cardiovascular endurance*. Unpublished honor's thesis, Sydney Teacher's College, Australia.

Rushall, B.S. (1965). Psychological factors in training. *International Swimmer*, **1**, 8-16.

Rushall, B.S. (1967a). A model for the psychological control of swimmers. *Journal of the British Swimming Coaches' Association*, **45**, 20-32.

Rushall, B.S. (1967b). Personality profiles and a theory of behavior modification. *Swimming Technique*, **4**, 66-76.

Rushall, B.S. (1967c). *The scientific bases of circulorespiratory endurance training*. Unpublished master's thesis, Indiana University, Bloomington.

Rushall, B.S. (1970a). An evaluation of the relationship between personality and physical performance categories. In G.S. Kenyon (Ed.), *Contemporary psychology of sport*. Chicago: Athletic Institute.

Rushall, B.S. (1970b). Some applications of psychology to swimming. *Swimming Technique, 7*, 71-82.

Rushall, B.S. (1971, October). *The environment as a significant source of variance in the study of personality.* Paper presented at the Third Canadian Psychomotor Learning and Sport Psychology Symposium, Vancouver, BC.

Rushall, B.S. (1974, October). *A tool for new directions in sport personality research: Behavior inventories for swimmers.* Paper presented at the Sixth Canadian Symposium for Psychomotor Learning and Sport Psychology, Halifax, NS.

Rushall, B.S. (1975a). Applied behavior analysis for sports and physical education. *International Journal of Sport Psychology, 6*, 75-88.

Rushall, B.S. (1975b). Applied psychology of sports. In B.S. Rushall (Ed.), *The status of psychomotor learning and sport psychology research.* Dartmouth, NS: Sports Science Associates.

Rushall, B.S. (1975c). Psychodynamics and personality in sport: Status and values. In H.T.A. Whiting (Ed.), *Readings in sport psychology* (pp. 72-84). London: Lepus Books.

Rushall, B.S. (1975d). Psycho-social factors in performance. In J. Taylor (Ed.), *Science and the athlete.* Ottawa, ON: Coaching Association of Canada.

Rushall, B.S. (1978a). The bases for advocating applied behavior analysis as a psychology for practitioners. In D.M. Landers & R.W. Christina (Eds.), *Psychology of motor behavior and sport—1977* (pp. 284-298). Champaign, IL: Human Kinetics.

Rushall, B.S. (1978b). Environment specific behavior inventories: Developmental procedures. *International Journal of Sport Psychology, 9*, 97-110.

Rushall, B.S. (1979). *Psyching in sport.* London: Pelham Books.

Rushall, B.S. (1980). Using applied behavior analysis for altering motivation. In R.M. Suinn (Ed.), *Psychology in sports: Methods and applications* (pp. 63-72). Minneapolis: Burgess.

Rushall, B.S. (1982). The content of competition thinking—strategies. In L. Wankel & R.B. Wilberg (Eds.), *Psychology of sport and motor behavior: Research and practice.* Edmonton: University of Alberta.

Rushall, B.S. (1984). The content of competition thinking. In W.F. Straub & J.M. Williams (Eds.), *Cognitive sport psychology.* Lansing, NY: Sport Science Associates.

Rushall, B.S. (1985a). The effects of three selected cognitive patterns on rowing ergometer performance. In J. Albinson (Ed.), *Proceedings of the 1984 annual symposium of the Canadian Society for Psychomotor Learning and Sport Psychology.* Kingston, ON: Queen's University.

Rushall, B.S. (1985b). *The sport psychology consultation system.* Spring Valley, CA: Sports Science Associates.

Rushall, B.S. (1986). *The psychology of successful cross-country ski racing.* Ottawa, ON: Cross Country Canada.

Rushall, B.S. (1992). *Mental skills training for sports.* Spring Valley, CA: Sports Science Associates.

Rushall, B.S., & Fry, D. (1980). Behavior variables in superior swimmers. *Canadian Journal of Applied Sport Sciences,* **5,** 177-182.

Rushall, B.S., & Leet, D. (1979). An assessment of the prediction of swimming performance in competition from behavioral information. *Canadian Journal of Applied Sport Sciences,* **4,** 154-157.

Rushall, B.S., & MacEachern, J.A. (1977). The effects of systematic behavioral feedback on teaching behaviors of student physical education teachers. *Canadian Journal of Applied Sport Sciences,* **2,** 161-169.

Rushall, B.S., & Siedentop, D. (1972). *The development and control of behavior in sport and physical education.* Philadelphia: Lea & Febiger.

Rushall, B.S., & Smith, K.C. (1979). The modification of the quality and quantity of behavior categories in a swimming coach. *Journal of Sport Psychology,* **1,** 138-150.

Ryan, E.D. (1961). Motor performance under stress as a function of practice. *Perceptual and Motor Skills,* **13,** 103-106.

Ryan, E.D. (1981). The emergence of psychological research as related to performance in physical activity. In G.A. Brooks (Ed.), *Perspectives on the academic discipline of physical education* (pp. 327-341). Champaign, IL: Human Kinetics.

Safrit, M.J., & Patterson, P. (1986). *Research Quarterly for Exercise and Sport* survey. *Research Quarterly for Exercise and Sport,* **57,** 91-100.

Salazar, W., Landers, D.M., Petruzzello, S.J., Crews, D.J., & Kubitz, K.A. (1988). The effects of physical/cognitive load on electrocortical patterns preceding response execution in archery. *Psychophysiology,* **25,** 478-479.

Salmela, J.H. (1979). Psychology and sport: Fear of applying. In P. Klavora & J.V. Daniel (Eds.), *Coach, athlete and the sport psychologist* (pp. 13-21). Toronto, ON: University of Toronto.

Salmela, J.H. (1981). *The world sport psychology sourcebook.* Ithaca, NY: Mouvement.

Salmela, J.H. (1984). Comparative sport psychology. In J.M. Silva & R.S. Weinberg (Eds.), *Psychological foundations of sport* (pp. 23-34). Champaign, IL: Human Kinetics.

Sanderson, F.H., & Whiting, H.T.A. (1978). Dynamic visual acuity as a predictive factor in ball-catching task. *Journal of Motor Behavior,* **10,** 107-114.

Sarason, S.B., Hill, K.T., & Zimbardo, P.G. (1964). A longitudinal study of the relation of test anxiety to performance on intelligence and achievement tests. *Monographs of the Society for Research in Child Development,* (Serial No. 9829, Whole No. 7).

Schlipp, P.A. (Ed.) (1951). *Albert Einstein.* New York: Harper.

Schmidt, R.A. (1975). A schema theory of discrete motor skill learning. *Psychological Review,* **82,** 225-260.

Schmidt, R.A. (1980). Past and future issues in motor programming. *Research Quarterly for Exercise and Sport*, **51**, 122-140.

Schmidt, R.A. (1985). The search for invariance in skilled movement behavior. *Research Quarterly for Exercise and Sport*, **56**, 188-200.

Schmidt, R.A. (1988). *Motor control and learning: A behavioral emphasis* (2nd ed.). Champaign, IL: Human Kinetics.

Schoenfeld, A.H., & Herrmann, D.J. (1982). Problem perception and knowledge structure in expert and novice mathematical problem solvers. *Journal of Experimental Psychology: Learning, Memory and Cognition*, **8**, 484-494.

Scholz, J.P., Kelso, J.A.S., & Schöner, G. (1987). Nonequilibrium phase transitions in coordinated biological motion: Critical slowing down and switching time. *Physics Letters A*, **123**, 390-394.

Schöner, G., Haken, H., & Kelso, J.A.S. (1986). A stochastic theory of phase transitions in human hand movement. *Biological Cybernetics*, **53**, 247-257.

Schöner, G., & Kelso, J.A.S. (1988a). A synergetic theory of environmentally-specified and learned patterns of movement coordination: I. Relative phase dynamics. *Biological Cybernetics*, **58**, 71-80.

Schöner, G., & Kelso, J.A.S. (1988b). A synergetic theory of environmentally-specified and learned patterns of movement coordination: II. Component oscillator dynamics. *Biological Cybernetics*, **58**, 81-89.

Schöner, G., & Kelso, J.A.S. (1988c). Dynamic pattern generation in behavioral and neural systems. *Science*, **239**, 1513-1520.

Schutz, R.W., & Gessaroli, M.E. (1987). The analysis of repeated measures designs involving multiple dependent variables. *Research Quarterly for Exercise and Sport*, **58**, 132-149.

Schutz, W.C. (1966). *The interpersonal underworld* (5th ed.). Palo Alto, CA: Science and Behavior Books.

Schutz, W.C. (1967). *The FIRO scales*. Palo Alto, CA: Consulting Psychologist Press.

Scriven, M. (1972). Objectivity and subjectivity in educational research. In L.B. Thomas (Ed.), *Philosophical redirection of educational research*. Chicago: University of Chicago Press.

Seefeldt, V., & Haubenstricker, J. (1982). Patterns, phases, or stages: An analytical model for the study of developmental movement. In J.A.S. Kelso & J.E. Clark (Eds.), *The development of movement control and coordination* (pp. 309-318). Chichester, UK: Wiley.

Selkirk, R.V. (1980). *The effects of cognitive strategies on running performance*. Unpublished master's thesis, Lakehead University, Thunder Bay, ON.

Selverston, A.I. (1980). Are central pattern generators understandable? *The Behavioral and Brain Sciences*, **3**, 535.

Shannon, C.E., & Weaver, W. (1949). *The mathematical theory of communication*. Urbana: University of Illinois Press.

Sharp, R.H., & Whiting, H.T.A. (1974). Exposure and occluded duration effects on ball-catching skill. *Journal of Motor Behavior*, **6**, 139-148.

Sherrington, C.S. (1906). *The integrative action of the nervous system*. New Haven, CT: Yale University Press.

Sherrington, C.S. (1940). *Man on his nature*. Cambridge, UK: Cambridge University Press.

Shewchuk, M. (1985). *Aspects of thought factors and their effects on performance in swimming*. Unpublished master's thesis, Lakehead University, Thunder Bay, ON.

Shuttleworth, F.K. (1939). The physical and mental growth of girls and boys age six to nineteen in relation to age at maximum growth. *Monographs of the Society for Research in Child Development*, **4**(3, serial no. 22).

Siegal, M.H., & Zeigler, H.P. (Eds.) (1976). *Psychological research: The inside story*. New York: Harper & Row.

Silva, J.M., & Weinberg, R.S. (Eds.) (1984). *Psychological foundations of sport*. Champaign, IL: Human Kinetics.

Simon, R.J. (1974). The work habits of eminent scientists. *Sociology of Work and Occupations*, **1**, 327-335.

Simonton, D.K. (1984). *Genius, creativity, and leadership*. Cambridge, MA: Harvard University Press.

Simonton, D.K. (1987). Developmental antecedents of achieved eminence. *Annals of Child Development*, **5**, 131-169.

Simonton, D.K. (1988). *Scientific genius: A psychology of science*. Cambridge, UK: Cambridge University Press.

Simonton, D.K. (1989). Chance-configuration theory of scientific creativity. In B. Gholson, W.R. Shadish, Jr., R.A. Neimeyer, & A.C. Houts (Eds.), *Psychology of science: Contributions to metascience* (pp. 170-213). Cambridge, UK: Cambridge University Press.

Singer, R.N. (1968). *Motor learning and human performance*. New York: Macmillan.

Singer, R.N. (1972). *Coaching, athletics, and psychology*. New York: McGraw-Hill.

Singer, R.N. (1978a). Motor skills and learning strategies. In H.F. O'Neil, Jr. (Ed.), *Learning strategies*. New York: Academic Press.

Singer, R.N. (1978b). The readiness to learn skills necessary for participation in sport. In R.A. Magill, M.A. Ash, & F.L. Smoll (Eds.), *Children in sport: A contemporary anthology* (pp. 29-39). Champaign, IL: Human Kinetics.

Singer, R.N. (1980). Motor behavior and the role of cognitive processes and learner strategies. In G.E. Stelmach & J. Requin (Eds.), *Tutorials in motor behavior*. Amsterdam: North-Holland.

Singer, R.N. (1982). *The learning of motor skills*. New York: Macmillan.

Singer, R.N. (1984). *Sustaining motivation in sport*. Tallahassee, FL: Sport Consultants International.

Singer, R.N. (1986). *Peak performance . . . and more*. Ithaca, NY: Mouvement.

Singer, R.N. (1990). Motor learning research: Meaningful for physical educators or a waste of time? *Quest*, **42**, 114-125.

Singer, R.N., & Gerson, R.F. (1981). Task classification and strategy utilization in motor skills. *Research Quarterly for Exercise and Sport*, **52**, 100-116.

Singer, R.N., DeFrancesco, C., & Randall, L.E. (1989). Effectiveness of a global learning strategy practiced in different contexts on primary and transfer self-paced motor tasks. *Journal of Sport and Exercise Psychology*, **11**, 290-303.

Singer, R.N., Flora, L.A., & Abourezk, T.L. (1989). The effect of a five-step cognitive learning strategy on the acquisition of a complex motor skill. *Journal of Applied Sport Psychology*, **1**, 98-108.

Singer, R.N., Hagenbeck, F., & Gerson, R.F. (1981). Strategy enhancement of serial motor skill acquisition. *Bulletin of the Psychonomic Society*, **18**, 148-150.

Singer, R.N., & McCaughan, L.R. (1978). Motivational effects of attributions, expectancy, and achievement motivation during the learning of a novel motor task. *Journal of Motor Behavior*, **10**, 245-254.

Singer, R.N., & Suwanthada, S. (1986). The generalizability effectiveness of a learning strategy on achievement in related closed motor skills. *Research Quarterly for Exercise and Sport*, **57**, 205-213.

Skinner, B.F. (1938). *The behavior of organisms*. New York: Appleton-Century-Crofts.

Skinner, B.F. (1950). Are theories of learning necessary? *Psychological Review*, **57**, 193-216.

Skinner, B.F. (1956). A case history in scientific method. *American Psychologist*, **2**, 221-233.

Skinner, B.F. (1983). *A matter of consequences*. New York: Knopff.

Smart, R.G. (1964). The importance of negative results in psychological research. *Canadian Psychologist*, **5**, 225-232.

Smoll, F.L. (1982). Developmental kinesiology: Toward a subdiscipline focusing on motor development. In J.A.S. Kelso & J.E. Clark (Eds.), *The development of movement control and co-ordination* (pp. 319-354). Chichester, UK: Wiley.

Snyder, C.W., Jr., & Abernethy, B. (1991). *Experimental inquiry*. Unpublished manuscript.

Snyder, C.W., Jr., & Law, H.G. (1979). Three-mode common factor analysis: Procedure and computer programs. *Multivariate Behavioral Research*, **14**, 435-441.

Spilich, G.J., Vesonder, G.T., Chiesi, H.L., & Voss, J.F. (1979). Text processing of individuals with high and low domain knowledge. *Journal of Verbal Learning and Verbal Behavior*, **18**, 275-290.

Spink, K.S., & Roberts, G.C. (1980). Ambiguity of outcome and causal attributions. *Journal of Sport Psychology*, **23**, 237-244.

Spirduso, W.W. (1981). The emergence of research in motor control and learning. In G.A. Brooks (Ed.), *Perspectives on the academic discipline of physical education* (pp. 255-272). Champaign, IL: Human Kinetics.

Spitz, H.H. (1966). The role of input organization in the learning and memory of mental retardates. In N.R. Ellis (Ed.), *International review of research in mental retardation* (Vol. 2). New York: Academic Press.

Stelmach, G.E. (1987). The cutting edge of research in physical education and exercise science: The search for understanding. In M.J. Safrit & H.M. Eckert (Eds.), *The cutting edge in physical education and exercise science research* (pp. 8-25). Champaign, IL: Human Kinetics.

Stelmach, G.E., & Diggles, V.A. (1982). Control theories in motor behavior. *Acta Psychologica, 50,* 83-105.

Stelmach, G.E., & Kelso, J.A.S. (1973). Distance and location cues in short-term motor memory. *Perceptual and Motor Skills, 37,* 403-406.

Stelmach, G.E., & Kelso, J.A.S. (1975). Memory trace strength and response biasing in short-term memory. *Memory and Cognition, 3,* 58-62.

Stelmach, G.E., Kelso, J.A.S., & Wallace, S.A. (1975). Preselection in short-term memory. *Journal of Experimental Psychology: Human Learning and Memory, 1,* 745-755.

Sternberg, S. (1969). The discovery of processing stages: Extensions of Donder's method. In W.G. Koster (Ed.), *Attention and Performance II. Acta Psychologica, 30,* 276-315.

Stott, D.H., Moyes, F.A., & Henderson, S.E. (1984). *Manual: Test of motor impairment (Henderson revision).* Guelph, Netherlands: Brook Educational.

Stratton, R.K. (1977). *Developmental aspects of attention in motor skill performance of children.* Unpublished doctoral dissertation, Florida State University, Tallahassee.

Straub, William F. (Ed.). (1991). *Sport Psychology: An Analysis of Athlete Behavior* (2nd ed.). Longmeadow, MA: Mouvement.

Sugden, D.A. (1978). Visual motor short term memory in educationally subnormal boys. *British Journal of Educational Psychology, 48,* 330-339.

Sugden, D.A. (1980a). Developmental strategies in motor and visual short term memory. *Perceptual and Motor Skills, 51,* 146.

Sugden, D.A. (1980b). Movement speed in children. *Journal of Motor Behavior, 12,* 125-132.

Sugden, D.A. (1986). The development of proprioception. In H.T.A. Whiting & M.G. Wade (Eds.), *Themes in motor development* (pp. 21-40). Dordrecht, Netherlands: Martinus Nijhoff.

Sugden, D.A. (1990). The role of proprioception in eye hand coordination. In C. Bard, M. Fleury, & L. Hay (Eds.), *Development of eye hand coordination across the lifespan* (pp. 133-153). Columbia: University of South Carolina.

Sugden, D.A., & Gray, S.D.M. (1981). Capacities, strategies and movement speed of educational subnormal boys of serial and discrete motor skills. *British Journal of Educational Psychology, 51,* 77-82.

Sugden, D.A., & Keogh, J.F. (1990). *Problems in movement skill development.* Columbia: University of South Carolina Press.

Sugden, D.A., & Newall, M. (1987). Teaching transfer strategies to children with moderate learning difficulties. *British Journal of Special Education,* **14**(2), 63-67.

Sugden, D.A., & Wann, C. (1987). The assessment of motor impairment in children with moderate learning difficulties. *British Journal of Educational Psychology,* **57**, 225-236.

Summers, J.J., & Ford, S.K. (1990). The test of attentional and interpersonal style: An evaluation. *International Journal of Sport Psychology,* **21**, 102-111.

Taylor, J.A. (1953). A personality scale of manifest anxiety. *Journal of Abnormal and Social Psychology,* **48**, 285-290.

Thelen, E. (1985). Developmental origins of motor coordination: Leg movements in human infants. *Developmental Psychobiology,* **18**, 1-22.

Thelen, E. (1986). Development of coordinated movement: Implications for early human development. In M.G. Wade & H.T.A. Whiting (Eds.), *Motor development in children: Aspects of coordination and control* (pp. 107-124). Dordrecht, Netherlands: Martinus Nijhoff.

Thelen, E. (1989). The (re)discovery of motor development: Learning new things from an old field. *Developmental Psychology,* **25**, 946-949.

Thelen, E., Kelso, J.A.S., & Fogel, A. (1987). Self-organizing systems and infant motor development. *Developmental Review,* **7**, 39-65.

Thelen, E., Skala, K.D., & Kelso, J.A.S. (1987). The dynamic nature of early coordination: Evidence from bilateral leg movements in young infants. *Developmental Psychology,* **23**, 179-186.

Thomas, J.R. (1977a). A note concerning analysis of error scores from motor memory research. *Journal of Motor Behavior,* **9**, 251-253.

Thomas, J.R. (1977b). *Youth sport guide for coaches and parents.* Washington, DC: American Alliance for Health, Physical Education, and Recreation.

Thomas, J.R. (1980). Acquisition of motor skills: Information processing differences between children and adults. *Research Quarterly for Exercise and Sport,* **51**, 158-173.

Thomas, J.R. (Ed.) (1984). *Motor development during childhood and adolescence.* Minneapolis: Burgess.

Thomas, J.R. (1985). Physical education and paranoia—Synonyms. *Journal of Physical Education, Recreation and Dance,* **56**, 20-22.

Thomas, J.R. (1987a). Are we already in pieces, or just falling apart? *Quest,* **39**, 114-121.

Thomas, J.R. (1987b). 7 ± 2: Miller must have been an assistant professor. *Perceptual and Motor Skills,* **64**, 1285-1286.

Thomas, J.R. (1989). Naturalistic research can drive motor development theory. In J.S. Skinner, C.B. Corbin, D.M. Landers, P.E. Martin, &

C.L. Wells (Eds.), *Future directions in exercise and sport science research* (pp. 349-367). Champaign, IL: Human Kinetics.

Thomas, J.R. (1990). The body of knowledge: A common core. In C. Corbin & H.M. Eckert (Eds.), *The evolving undergraduate major.* Champaign, IL: Human Kinetics.

Thomas, J.R. (1991). Studying human movement: Research questions should drive assignment of labels. In R.J. Park & H.M. Eckert (Eds.), *The Academy papers: New possibilities, new paradigms?* (pp. 115-121). Champaign, IL: Human Kinetics.

Thomas, J.R., & Bender, P.R. (1977). A developmental explanation for children's motor behavior: A neo-Piagetian interpretation. *Journal of Motor Behavior, 9*, 81-93.

Thomas, J.R., & Chissom, B.S. (1972). Relationships as assessed by canonical correlation between perceptual-motor and intellectual abilities for pre-school and early elementary age children. *Journal of Motor Behavior, 4*, 23-29.

Thomas, J.R., & Chissom, B.S. (1974a). Prediction of first grade academic performance from kindergarten perceptual-motor data. *Research Quarterly, 45*, 148-153.

Thomas, J.R., & Chissom, B.S. (1974b). Relationships among perceptual-motor measures and their correlations with academic readiness for preschool children. *Perceptual and Motor Skills, 39*, 467-473.

Thomas, J.R., Chissom, B.S., & Biasiotto, J. (1972). Investigation of the Shape-O Ball Test as a perceptual-motor task for pre-schoolers. *Perceptual and Motor Skills, 35*, 447-450.

Thomas, J.R., Chissom, B.S., Stewart, C., & Shelley, F. (1975). Effects of perceptual-motor training on pre-school children: A multivariate approach. *Research Quarterly, 46*, 505-513.

Thomas, J.R., & French, K.E. (1984). *Gender differences in motor performance: A meta-analysis.* Paper presented at the annual meeting of the American Alliance for Health, Physical Education, Recreation and Dance, Anaheim, California.

Thomas, J.R., & French, K.E. (1985). Gender differences across age in motor performance: A meta-analysis. *Psychological Bulletin, 98*, 260-282.

Thomas, J.R., & French, K.E. (1986). The use of meta-analysis in exercise and sport. *Research Quarterly for Exercise and Sport, 57*, 196-204.

Thomas, J.R., French, K.E., & Humphries, C.A. (1986). Knowledge development and sport skill performance: Directions for motor behavior research. *Journal of Sport Psychology, 8*, 259-272.

Thomas, J.R., French, K.E., Thomas, K.T., & Gallagher, J.D. (1988). Children's knowledge development and sport performance. In F.L. Smoll, M. Ash, & R. Magill (Eds.), *Children in sport, 3rd ed.* (pp. 179-202). Champaign, IL: Human Kinetics.

Thomas, J.R., & Gallagher, J.D. (1986). Memory development and skill acquisition. In V. Seefeldt (Ed.), *Physical activity and well-being* (pp. 127-139). Reston, VA: American Alliance for Health, Physical Education, Recreation and Dance.

Thomas, J.R., Lee, A.M., & Thomas, K.T. (1988a). *Physical education for children: Concepts into practice.* Champaign, IL: Human Kinetics.

Thomas, J.R., Lee, A.M., & Thomas, K.T. (1988b). *Physical education for children: Daily lesson plans.* Champaign, IL: Human Kinetics.

Thomas, J.R., & Marzke, M.W. (1992). The development of gender differences in throwing: Is human evolution a factor? In R.W. Christina and H.M. Eckert (Eds.), *The Academy papers: Enhancing human performance in sport.* Champaign, IL: Human Kinetics.

Thomas, J.R., Mitchell, B., & Solmon, M.A. (1979). Precision knowledge of results and motor performance: Relationship to age. *Research Quarterly, 50,* 687-698.

Thomas, J.R., & Moon, D. (1976). Measuring motor rhythmic ability in children. *Research Quarterly, 47,* 20-32.

Thomas, J.R., & Nelson, J.K. (1985). *Introduction to research in health, physical education, recreation and dance.* Champaign, IL: Human Kinetics.

Thomas, J.R., & Nelson, J.K. (1990). *Research methods in physical activity.* Champaign, IL: Human Kinetics.

Thomas, J.R., & Nelson, J.K. (1991). A developmental analysis of gender differences in health related physical fitness. *Pediatric Exercise Science, 3,* 28-42.

Thomas, J.R., Pierce, C., & Ridsdale, S. (1977). Age differences in children's ability to model motor behavior. *Research Quarterly, 48,* 592-597.

Thomas, J.R., Salazar, W., & Landers, D.M. (1991). What is missing in $p < .05$? Effect size. *Research Quarterly for Exercise and Sport, 62,* 344-348.

Thomas, J.R., & Stratton, R.K. (1977). Effect of divided attention on children's rhythmic response. *Research Quarterly, 48,* 428-435.

Thomas, J.R., & Thomas, K.T. (1986). The relation of movement and cognitive function. In V. Seefeldt (Ed.), *Physical activity and well-being* (pp. 443-452). Reston, VA: American Alliance for Health, Physical Education, Recreation and Dance.

Thomas, J.R., & Thomas, K.T. (1987). [Review of *The physical side of thinking*]. *Journal of Physical Education, Recreation and Dance, 58*(4), 82-85.

Thomas, J.R., & Thomas, K.T. (1988). Development of gender differences in physical activity. *Quest, 40,* 219-229.

Thomas, J.R., & Thomas, K.T. (1989). What is motor development: Where does it belong? *Quest, 41,* 203-212.

Thomas, J.R., Thomas, K.T., Lee, A.M., Testerman, E., & Ashy, A. (1983). Age differences in use of strategy for recall of movement in a large scale environment. *Research Quarterly for Exercise and Sport, 54,* 264-272.

Thomas, K.T. (1981). *Age differences in memory for movement: Effects of strategy and preselection when ecological validity is varied.* Unpublished doctoral dissertation, Louisiana State University, Baton Rouge.

Thomas, K.T., & Thomas, J.R. (1988). Perceptual development and its differential influence on limb positioning under two movement conditions in children. In J.E. Clark & J.H. Humphrey (Eds.), *Advances in motor development* (Vol. 2). New York: AMS Press.

Thorndike, E.L. (1914). *Educational psychology*. New York: Columbia University.

Thurstone, L.L. (1935). *Vectors of the mind*. Chicago: University of Chicago Press.

Tolman, E.C. (1932). *Purposive behavior in animals and men*. New York: Appleton-Century-Crofts.

Toulman, S. (1958). *The uses of argument*. Cambridge, UK: Cambridge University Press.

Triplett, N. (1898). The dynamogenic factors in pacemaking and competition. *American Journal of Psychology*, **9**, 507-553.

Tuddenham, R.D., & Snyder, M.M. (1954). Physical growth of California boys and girls from birth to 18 years. *Child Development*, **1**, 183-364.

Tuller, B., & Kelso, J.A.S. (1984). The timing of articulatory gestures: Evidence for relational invariants. *Journal of the Acoustical Society of America*, **76**(4), 1030-1036.

Tuller, B., & Kelso, J.A.S. (1985). *Coordination in normal and split-brain patients*. Paper presented at the meeting of the Psychonomic Society, Boston.

Tuller, B., Kelso, J.A.S., & Harris, K.S. (1982). Interarticulator phasing as an index of temporal regularity in speech. *Journal of Experimental Psychology: Human Perception and Performance*, **8**, 460-472.

Tuller, B., Kelso, J.A.S., & Harris, K.S. (1983). Converging sources of evidence of relative timing in speech production. *Journal of Experimental Psychology: Human Perception and Performance*, **9**, 829-833.

Turvey, M.T. (1977). Preliminaries to a theory of action with reference to vision. In R. Shaw & J. Bransford (Eds.), *Perceiving, acting and knowing* (pp. 211-263). Hillsdale, NJ: Erlbaum.

Turvey, M.T., & Carello, C. (1986). The ecological approach to perceiving-acting: A pictorial essay. *Acta Psychologica*, **63**, 133-155.

Turvey, M.T., & Carello, C. (1988). Exploring a law-based ecological approach to skilled action. In A.M. Colley & J.R. Beech (Eds.), *Cognition and action in skilled behaviour* (pp. 191-203). Amsterdam: North-Holland.

Tussing, L. (1940). The effects of football and basketball on vision. *Research Quarterly*, **11**, 16-18.

Tyldesley, D.A., & Whiting, H.T.A. (1975). Operational timing. *Journal of Human Movement Studies*, **1**, 172-177.

Ulrich, C. (1957). Measurement of stress evidenced by college women in situations involving competition. *Research Quarterly*, **28**, 160-172.

Unestahl, L.-E. (Ed.) (1983). *The mental aspects of gymnastics*. Orebro, Sweden: Veje Forlag.

Vallery-Radot, R. (1911). *The life of Pasteur* (R.S. Devonshire, Trans.). London, UK: Constable.

van Wieringen, P.C.W., & Bootsma, R.J. (1989). *Catching up: Selected essays of H.T.A. Whiting*. Amsterdam: Free University Press.

Wade, M.G. (1976). Developmental motor learning. *Exercise and Sport Sciences Reviews*, **4**, 375-394.

Wade, M.G., & Whiting, H.T.A. (1986). *Motor development in children: Aspects of coordination and control*. Dordrecht, Netherlands: Martinus Nijhoff.

Wall, A.E. (1986). A knowledge-based approach to motor skill acquisition. In M.G. Wade & H.T.A. Whiting (Eds.), *Motor development in children: Aspects of coordination and control* (pp. 33-49). Dordrecht, Netherlands: Martinus Nijhoff.

Wall, A.E., McClements, J., Bouffard, M., Findlay, H., & Taylor, M.J. (1985). A knowledge-based approach to motor development: Implications for the physically awkward. *Adapted Physical Activity Quarterly*, **2**, 21-42.

Wallace, S.A., De Oreo, K.L., & Roberts, G.C. (1976). Memory and perceptual trace development in ballistic timing. *Journal of Motor Behavior*, **8**, 133-137.

Weimer, W.B., & Palermo, D.S. (1973). Paradigms and normal science in psychology. *Science Studies*, **3**, 211-244.

Weiner, B. (1972). *Theories of motivation: From mechanism to cognition*. Chicago, IL: Markham.

Weiner, B., Frieze, S., Kukla, A., Reed, L., Rest, C., & Rosenbaum, R.M. (1971). *Perceiving the causes of success and failure*. New York: General Learning Press.

Weiss, P. (November, 1969). Living nature and the knowledge gap. *Saturday Review*, **52**(48), 19-22, 56.

White, R.K. (1931). The versality of genius. *Journal of Social Psychology*, **2**, 460-489.

Whiting, H.T.A. (1967). *Visual motor coordination*. Unpublished doctoral dissertation, University of Leeds, UK.

Whiting, H.T.A. (1969). *Acquiring ball skill: A psychological interpretation*. London: Bell.

Whiting, H.T.A. (1970). *Teaching the persistent non-swimmer*. London: Bell.

Whiting, H.T.A. (Ed.) (1972). *Readings in sport psychology*. London: Kimpton.

Whiting, H.T.A. (1975a). *Concepts in skill learning*. London: Lepus Books.

Whiting, H.T.A. (1975b). Editorial. *Journal of Human Movement Studies*, **1**, 1-4.

Whiting, H.T.A. (Ed.) (1975c). *Readings in human performance*. London: Lepus Books.

Whiting, H.T.A. (Ed.) (1975d). *Readings in sport psychology 2*. London: Kimpton.

Whiting, H.T.A. (1980). Dimension of control in motor learning. In G.E. Stelmach & J. Requin (Eds.), *Tutorials in motor behavior* (pp. 537-550). Amsterdam: North-Holland.

Whiting, H.T.A. (1982). Skill in sport—a descriptive and prescriptive appraisal. In J.H. Salmela, J.T. Partington, & T. Orlick (Eds.), *New paths of sport learning and excellence* (pp. 7-13). Ottawa, ON: Sport in Perspective.

Whiting, H.T.A. (Ed.) (1984). *Human motor actions: Bernstein reassessed.* Amsterdam: Elsevier.

Whiting, H.T.A., & Cockerill, I.M. (1972). The development of a simple ballistic skill with and without visual control. *Journal of Motor Behavior*, **4**, 155-162.

Whiting, H.T.A., Gill, E.G., & Stephenson, J.M. (1970). Critical time intervals for taking in flight information in a ball-catching task. *Ergonomics*, **13**, 265-272.

Whiting, H.T.A., & Wade, M.G. (Eds.) (1986). *Themes in motor development.* Dordrecht, Netherlands: Martinus Nijhoff.

Whitson, D.J. (1978). Sociology, psychology and Canadian sport. *Canadian Journal of Applied Sport Sciences*, **3**, 71-78.

Widmeyer, W.N., Brawley, L.R., & Carron, A.V. (1985). *The measurement of cohesion in sport teams.* London, ON: Sports Dynamics.

Wiener, N. (1948). *Cybernetics.* New York: Wiley.

Wiggins, D.K. (1984). The history of sport psychology in North America. In J.M. Silva & R.S. Weinberg (Eds.), *Psychological foundations of sport* (pp. 274-286). Champaign, IL: Human Kinetics.

Wilberg, R.B. (1972). A suggested direction for the study of motor performance by physical educators. *Research Quarterly*, **43**, 387-393.

Winther, K.T., & Thomas, J.R. (1981). Developmental differences in children's labeling of movement. *Journal of Motor Behavior*, **13**, 77-90.

Woodworth, R.S. (1899). The accuracy of voluntary movement. *Psychological Review*, **3**(Suppl. 2).

Woodworth, R.S. (1903). *Le mouvement.* Paris: Doin.

Woodworth, R.S. (1938). *Experimental psychology.* New York: Holt.

Wundt, W. (1907). *Outlines of psychology* (C.J. Judd, Trans.). Leipzig, Germany: Engelmann.

Yamanishi, T., Kawato, J., & Suzuki, R. (1980). Two coupled oscillators as a model for the coordinated finger tapping by both hands. *Biological Cybernetics*, **37**, 219-225.

Zahar, E. (1973). Why did Einstein's programme supersede Lorentz's? *British Journal for the Philosophy of Science*, **24**, 95-123, 223-263.

Zanone, P.G., & Hauert, C.A. (1987). For a cognitive conception of motor processes: A provocative standpoint. *European Bulletin of Cognitive Psychology*, **7**(2), 109-129.

Zuckerman, H.A. (1975). *Scientific elite: Studies of Nobel laureates in the United States.* Chicago: University of Chicago Press.

Zuckerman, H.A., & Merton, R.K. (1971). Patterns of evaluation in science: Institutionalisation, structure and functions of the referee system. *Minerva*, **9**, 66-100.

Index